The Face

The Face
A Cultural History

FAY BOUND-ALBERTI

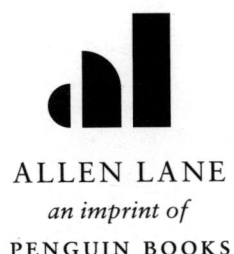

ALLEN LANE
an imprint of
PENGUIN BOOKS

ALLEN LANE

UK | USA | Canada | Ireland | Australia
India | New Zealand | South Africa

Allen Lane is part of the Penguin Random House group of companies
whose addresses can be found at global.penguinrandomhouse.com

Penguin Random House UK
One Embassy Gardens, 8 Viaduct Gardens, London SW11 7BW

penguin.co.uk

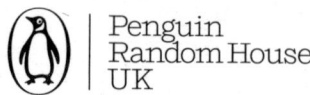

First published in Great Britain by Allen Lane 2026
001

Copyright © Fay Bound-Alberti, 2026

Penguin Random House values and supports copyright.
Copyright fuels creativity, encourages diverse voices, promotes freedom
of expression and supports a vibrant culture. Thank you for purchasing
an authorized edition of this book and for respecting intellectual property
laws by not reproducing, scanning or distributing any part of it by any
means without permission. You are supporting authors and enabling
Penguin Random House to continue to publish books for everyone.
No part of this book may be used or reproduced in any manner for the
purpose of training artificial intelligence technologies or systems. In accordance
with Article 4(3) of the DSM Directive 2019/790, Penguin Random House
expressly reserves this work from the text and data mining exception.

The moral right of the author has been asserted

Set in 12/14.75pt Dante MT Std
Typeset by Six Red Marbles UK, Thetford, Norfolk
Printed and bound in Great Britain by Clays Ltd, Elcograf S.p.A.

The authorized representative in the EEA is Penguin Random House Ireland,
Morrison Chambers, 32 Nassau Street, Dublin D02 YH68

A CIP catalogue record for this book is available from the British Library

ISBN: 978–0–241–67071–2

Penguin Random House is committed to a sustainable future
for our business, our readers and our planet. This book is made from
Forest Stewardship Council® certified paper.

*The face is the mirror of the mind,
and eyes without speaking confess the secrets of the heart.*

St Jerome

The face summons me to my obligations and judges me.

Emmanuel Levinas

*At 20 you have the face that nature gave you,
at 40 the face life gave you, and at 60 the face you deserve.*

Variously attributed

*To the faces I have loved and touched, yearned for and lost,
remembered, forgotten and failed to recognize.*

*To the faces I have known all their lives.
And to the faces I will never know.*

And to Millie and Jacob, whose faces I carry in my heart.

Contents

Acknowledgements	xi
Illustration Credits	xv
Introduction	xvii
1. Portrayed	1
2. Captured	37
3. Mirrored	66
4. Perfected	92
5. Grown	115
6. Expressed	137
7. Reconstructed	161
8. Recognized	185
9. Transplanted	208
Afterword	238
Index	245

Acknowledgements

In 2019 my life was changed by a UKRI Future Leaders Fellowship that made it possible for me to return to academia, and to research and write this book. Thanks to the panel members, reviewers and people whose work makes the Fellowship team so special – especially Kirsty Grainger, Steve Meader, Phil Edwards, Bridget Mellifont, Samantha Aspinall, Barry Smith and Paul Grimshaw.

I owe many personal debts – special thanks to Sandra Vigon for always lighting the way; to Louisa Young for making me a better writer, and to Patricia Greene and Paddy Ricard for always being on my side. For love and friendship, thanks to Mark Jenner, Emma Alberti, Karen Alberti, Ellen Bruno, Joanna Bourke, Caroline Edwards, Rana Baker, Dahlia Gubara, Erika Melek Delgado, Laura Gowing, Stephen Bound, Tiffany Watt-Smith, Alice Taylor, Anne Marie Rafferty, Heaven Crawley, Jacob Alberti, Erin Mawson, Millie Bound, Jon Ritchie, Alana Harris and Lina Khatib.

I have many colleagues at King's College London and the Digital Futures Institute to whom I am grateful – in particular, thanks to Marion Thain for inviting me to set up the Centre for Technology and the Body, to Simon Tanner, Paul Readman, Caitjan Gainty, Jonathan Gray, Simon Wessely, Jo Fitzpatrick, David Brydan, Kate Devlin, Jon Wilson, Stephen Lovell, Hannah Murphy and Richard Wingate.

For sharing their thoughts on art, science and facial reconstruction, thanks to Joe Mullins, Caroline Wilkinson, Oscar Nilsson, John Gurche, Lucy Burscough, Eleanor Crook, Stefanos Geroulanos and Helen Browell. For insights into portraiture, thanks to Ludmilla Jordanova, Philip Mould and Rosie Broadley, and into facial recognition, Rob Jenkins and Mike Burton. A special thank you to David Pitcher, for scanning my brain. Thanks to Mike Haas, for his dedication to the story of Isabelle Dinoire, and to the actors who have

Acknowledgements

shared their thoughts about faces: Adam Pearson, Sebastian Stan and Isabel Adomakoh-Young. I am grateful to Eleanor Walkington-Ellis and Kirsty Warner for their invaluable administrative support with Interface, and to Ricardo de Sao Joao for making opaque systems bearable. Thanks also to Alana Saad and Heather Wilson for archival and permissions support.

To the advisory board of Interface past and present, thank you, Manos Tsakiris, Joanna Zylinska, Anna Ciaunica, Richard Ashcroft, Karen Bloor, Alex Clarke, Antonia Cronin, Dan Glasier, Nichola Rumsey, Mandana Seyfeddinipur, Amanda Bates, Kathleen Bogart, Marc Crank, Jaz Gray, Graeme Heward, Phyllida Swift, and the late James Partridge.

A heartfelt thanks to those transplant recipients and family members who have been so generous with their time, especially Cor Hutton, Robert Chelsea, Carmen Tarleton, Joe DiMeo, Mitch Hunter, Dallas Wiens, Jessica DiMeo and Rose DiMeo, Annalyn Bell Wiens, Ebony Chelsea, Ricky Brown and Bill Preston. It has been an absolute privilege to get to know you all, and I am grateful for your trust and kindness. Sadly, Dallas and Mitch died before this book was published, so I'd like to remember them too.

In studying facial surgery and transplantation, I have acquired huge debts from all the surgeons and researchers who have shared their work, especially Bohdan Pomahac, Vijay Gorantla, Benedetto Longo, Simon Kay, David Leonard, Elena Tsangaris, Emily Herrington, Patrik Lassus, Nathalie Roche, Sheila Jowsey-Gregoire, Dan Saleh, Len Doyal, Henk Giele, Jim Benedict, Tim Mitchell, Peter Friend and the late Sir Peter Morris.

I am grateful to my literary agent, Adam Gauntlett at PFD, for listening to my ideas and championing this book, and to Laura Stickney, my commissioning editor at Penguin, for seeing its value. Thanks also to Kim Walker for taking on the baton, and for their help with images and copy-editing respectively, to Fahad Al-Amoudi and Richard Mason.

During the writing of this book, I was simultaneously creating a documentary to bring the stories of face-transplant patients to the

Acknowledgements

world. Both projects fed off one another and introduced a wonderful collaborative dimension to an act – writing – that is often so solitary. Thank you to George Carey, Alan Hayling and Robert Thirkell for helping me to understand the narrative art of film, to Lol Crawley, who may now be an Oscar winner, but will always be my little brother, and to my sister-in-law Annie Marter: thank you for your patience as I learned a new visual art. Thanks also to Paramount Studios for loaning their equipment; to James Erskine and Victoria Gregory at New Black Films for their advice, and to my crew and editors, especially Barry Gibb, Jeff Seelbach, Derrick Peters, Adam Laschinger, Scott Carrithers, Manuel Lopez, April Kirby, Hugh Williams, Scott Carrithers and Sam Billinge.

Finally, thank you reader, for choosing this book – whether it raises a smile or a frown, I hope it makes you think about the face a little differently.

Fay Bound-Alberti
London, July 2025

Illustration Credits

1. The Venus of Brassempouy, c. 25,000 BCE, dating from the Upper Palaeolithic period. © *Historic Images / Alamy Stock Photo*
2. Head of a Roman Patrician from Otricoli, c. 75–50 BCE. © *Steven Zucker*
3. Mummy portrait of Eirene, 50 CE. © *ARTGEN / Alamy Stock Photo*
4. Nicolaus of Prussia, *Saint Hedwig of Silesia*, 1353. *Public Domain*
5. Sir Thomas More (1478–1535), portrait painting by Hans Holbein the Younger, 1527. © *incamerastock / Alamy Stock Photo*
6. Leonardo da Vinci, *Mona Lisa*, c. 1503–19. *Creative Commons*
7. Albrecht Dürer, *Self-Portrait at Twenty-Eight*, 1500. *Creative Commons*
8. Diego Rodríguez de Silva y Velázquez, *Juan de Pareja*, c. 1650. © *MET/BOT / Alamy Stock Photo*
9. Frans Hals, *The Laughing Cavalier*, 1624, housed in The Wallace Collection. © *piemags / Alamy Stock Photo*
10. Eugène Delacroix, *Self-Portrait*, c. 1837. © *Art Collection 4 / Alamy Stock Photo*
11. Francis Bacon, *Study after Velázquez's Portrait of Pope Innocent X*, 1953. © *Artepics / Alamy Stock Photo*
12. Robert Cornelius, *Self-Portrait*, 1839. © *Bill Waterson / Alamy Stock Photo*
13. Alphonse Bertillon, mugshot of Francis Galton, 1893. © *Chronicle / Alamy Stock Photo*
14. Caravaggio, *Narcissus at the Fountain*, 1597–99. *Creative Commons*
15. Jan van Eyck, *The Arnolfini Portrait*, 1434. © *Artefact / Alamy Stock Photo*
16. Parmigianino, *Self-Portrait in a Convex Mirror*, c. 1524. © *Heritage Image Partnership Ltd / Alamy Stock Photo*
17. Joshua Reynolds, *Self-Portrait*, c. 1788. *Royal Collection Trust*

Illustration Credits

18. Johannes Gumpp, *Triple Self-Portrait*, 1646. © *Heritage Image Partnership Ltd / Alamy Stock Photo*
19. François Boucher, *Pompadour at Her Toilette*, 1750. © *President and Fellows of Harvard College*
20. Unknown artist, *The Puzzle of the Face*, 2024. *Creative Commons*
21. Lennart Nilsson, on the cover of *Life* magazine, 1965. *LENNART NILSSON, TT/SCIENCE PHOTO LIBRARY*
22. Lennart Nilsson, *Foetus at eighteen weeks*, 1965. *LENNART NILSSON, TT/SCIENCE PHOTO LIBRARY*
23. Giovanni Strazza, *The Veiled Virgin*, early 1850s. *Public Domain*
24. Chidiebere Ibe, a Black child *in utero*, 2021. © *Chidiebere ibe*
25. 'Laughter' Plate 10, Charles Le Brun, 1760. © *Well/BOT / Alamy Stock Photo*
26. Oscar Rejlander, 'Contempt', in Charles Darwin's *The Expression of the Emotions in Man and Animals*, 1872. © *akg-images*
27. Guillaume Duchenne and 'the old toothless man', 1862. © *The History Collection / Alamy Stock Photo*
28. Caroline Wilkinson, Reconstruction of Richard III, 2012. *Face Lab, Liverpool John Moores University*
29. Adrie and Alfons Kennis, the face of Shanidar Z, 2024. *Via Getty Images*
30. Bettmann / Bust of Prehistoric Man, 1908. *Via Getty Images*
31. Oscar Nilsson, *Gustav* (2006). © *Oscar Nilsson*
32. Oscar Nilsson, *Gertrude* (2023). © *Oscar Nilsson*
33. Unknown artist, *Richard III*, early 16th century portrait. © *Royal Collection Enterprises Limited 2025 | Royal Collection Trust*
34. 'This is a picture of your brain': an fMRI scan, 2022. *Courtesy of David Pitcher, University of York*
35. Lol Crawley, Robert Chelsea with his transplanted face, 2022. © *Fay Bound Alberti*
36. Lynn Johnson, Katie Stubblefield's new face, before transplant, 2017. © *Lynn Johnson*
37. Unknown artist, Mask of Agamemnon, c. 1500 BCE. © *Peter Eastland / Alamy Stock Photo*

Introduction

When I was four, I got lost on a beach in Conwy, North Wales. I was lost often as a child; left behind in markets and shopping centres, train stations and, once, on the ghost train of a visiting funfair.

On this occasion, I was found not by my family but by a friendly blonde stranger. She decided we would drive up and down the beachfront in search of my mother. I sat in the passenger seat with my legs stretched out, eating toffees from a bag she produced from the glove compartment. As we inched along the promenade, I scanned the faces of men, women and children who were buying candyfloss, roller-skating, shooting at targets. Those faces, looming in and out of view, were strange and incomprehensible to me: mouths open wide or broken into grins, eyes narrowed or crinkled at the corners. Nothing and nobody seemed familiar.

I was not concerned about the fact that I had lost my parents; I liked this new life of warm cars and bags of toffee. But then the driver pointed at a woman who was standing at the side of the road, peering in the windows of passing cars. 'Is that your mum?' she asked. I shrugged; I did not recognize the woman with dark hair who was waving at us. But then I saw that she was standing next to a taller man with fair hair, and a scowling girl, a little older than me, who was hanging onto the man's sleeve. A boy in a buggy sat between them, squirming as he tried to undo his harness. The pattern came into focus.

'Yes,' I said, reluctantly stuffing the toffees back into the glove compartment. 'That's her.'

Sometimes we research a topic thinking our motivation is intellectual, only later to realize its emotional origins. For twenty-five years I have researched the histories of medicine, emotion and the body, uncovering feelings like loneliness and love, wondering

Introduction

why hearts mattered so much to the Egyptians, or brains to the Victorians.

I had been studying faces for several years before I realized that day on the beach was not normal. Not the getting lost, though that happened to me more frequently than to most children, but the mystery of my own mother's face.

We all grow up thinking what we experience is normal, until we discover otherwise. There are no routine tests for prosopagnosia, or face-blindness, a condition where you can't hold in mind the association between a face and an individual person. Sometimes its onset is obvious and sudden: a head injury can turn spouses into strangers overnight. But most of the time prosopagnosia is something you grow up with, like left-handedness. Your facial blunders, moments of social awkwardness, are as baffling to you as to anyone else.

Given there is no cure for prosopagnosia, a diagnosis doesn't really enhance the quality of your life – but it can help colleagues to know why you walked past them on the street, and your boyfriend to understand why, at the movies, you helped yourself to another man's popcorn.

Such moments are embarrassing for one simple reason: we are expected to know people by their faces. While a face might change during a person's life – because of ageing, accident, illness, as much as fashion or lifestyle – it remains quintessentially theirs, the basis of their identity – personal, legal and social. Open your passport and there you are – staring out glumly, at least in British passports where smiles are not allowed. In some countries, including the U.S., you may smile in your passport photo, but your mouth must be closed and your eyes open. These images are subdued shadows of who we are in real life, but biometric snapshots contain and portray the precise facial measurements and configurations that make our faces, and therefore ourselves, uniquely identifiable.

Why and how did the face come to matter so much? And have its meanings changed? What difference does it make if you are 'bad with faces' when it comes to navigating the world around you? And how did the idea of ourselves, as specific named individuals with distinct and unique faces, come into being?

Today the idea that your face represents who you are seems obvious and natural – and yet what if I told you that for most of human history, people didn't think this way at all? What if the connection between faces and individual personhood – something we take for granted every time we unlock our phones with facial recognition, or pose for a selfie – is a relatively recent invention?

This book is a history of how that happened, and the seemingly simple equation we make between a single, unique face and a named individual. This connection, which I call 'facehood', has a history. Along the way the book explores the meanings of the face, in history and in the present, offering insights for our own well-being, and for the future.

We will see, as we trace the history of portraiture, and the ways in which the face has been imagined, understood, analysed and judged, that facehood was not inevitable but emerged from Western individualism, sparked by Renaissance humanism, to gather momentum in the centuries that followed.

Knowing the face, judging the face, comparing the face and classifying the face – things we all do today without thinking – are processes we learned from the Victorians, who learned them from the Renaissance, who learned them from the ancient Greeks and Romans. In imagining the face, each technological innovation, such as the camera, or social change, such as consumer capitalism, has reinvigorated earlier beliefs, and given them a modern twist. Even before the scientific myth of race, which prioritized white, Europeans faces, the colour of a person's face ranked them in a social hierarchy; and ideas about beauty were linked to morality in ways that determined a person's worth.

We judge everything about a person, from their race to their heredity, morality, emotional state, upbringing, social and even human value, just by looking at their face. How many hundreds, even thousands of decisions do we make every day based on how we feel about our face, and the faces of others? We presume that the face is an index to someone's trustworthiness, decency, morality. We rely on the face, and on received, internalized wisdom about the face, often subconsciously, in deciding whom to trust, befriend or marry, whom to avoid, what to buy, what financial risks to take, where to live, whom to care for. And the people we arrest, protect, condemn, or even kill – these decisions are influenced by their faces. Or rather, by our beliefs about those faces.

What happens if those judgements are flawed, and biased? And how do we know whether they are or not?

It's extraordinary, given the weight we assign to faces in everyday life, that we have largely studied their meanings in isolation from their historical context. We ask questions about race, identity and feeling, about facial fashions and aesthetics, we develop facial recognition and AI technologies, and we study histories of society and emotion as though the face is unchanging. We talk about human evolution as a product of language, without reference to facial appearance, expression or gesture, but how things are said and communicated are as important as what is said, when it comes to human interaction.

We have treated the face as something unchanging and ahistorical. We used to do that with emotions and bodies – before the 1990s when histories of both became mainstream, they were seen as culturally variable rather than cultural inventions. Now the histories of emotion and the body are broad and expansive, covering everything from tears to smiles, from hands to bowels.

Faces, too, are products of belief systems, languages and environments as much as they are skin, bone and muscle. And yet they have not received the same attention as emotions and bodies; somehow, we imagine that they sit outside of history, that they simply *are*, as plain as the nose on your face. This book changes that.

So, what is a human face? At the anatomical level the answer is relatively straightforward – eyes, nose, mouth, chin, cheekbones, eyebrows, ears, jawbone and brow, usually assembled in a broadly symmetrical manner. That anatomical structure gives clues to our evolution, as over time the face has flattened and shortened and adapted to our environment.

Introduction

Unlike those of chimpanzees, our closest living relative, human faces are integrated within the skull, rather than pushed out in front. And we have nearly twice as many facial muscles as chimps, facilitating far more complex emotional expressions. Beneath the skin, dozens of muscles and nerves work together to let us smile, chew, laugh, sing, talk, kiss – so many of the things that we associate with being human.

By Charles Darwin's time, our emotional expressions were coded and classified into standard types, following Renaissance thought. In the twenty-first century an almost identical version is used by the Federal Bureau of Investigation (FBI) to judge a person's guilt, so certain are we that facial expressions offer insights into an individual's psyche. As St Jerome put it, the face is 'the mirror of the mind'; it reveals exactly what a person is thinking and feeling. But is that really the case?

The story, as we'll discover, is more complex. We have layered the anatomy of the face – and what it does – with multiple meanings, some more tangible than others.

Faces are stamped on our passports to confirm our legal status, and on our hearts, when we think of those we love. We have developed a whole language of 'losing' and 'saving' face, which has more literal meanings for some people and some countries than others. Meanwhile, families and nations trace their ancestry down the line of an aquiline nose, a hooded eye, or a heavy brow. Faces can launch a thousand ships or function as sites of horror. Think of David's nocturnal transformation in the film *An American Werewolf in London* (1981), or Pennywise the clown with razor-sharp teeth and red eyes in Stephen King's novel *It* (1986).

Faces are not just visually important. When our facial anatomy is damaged, we lose functionality, and with it many things that we take for granted: eating and drinking without dribbling; opening and closing our eyes; kissing a loved one. This complex entanglement of emotional and physical factors is why the face is so special. It's also the only part of the human body where all our senses come together: smell, taste, sight, touch, hearing.

Introduction

Faces change over time, and in ways that reflect the lives we lead. As the saying goes (and the epigraph reads): 'At 20 you have the face that nature gave you, at 40 the face life gave you, and at 60 the face you deserve.'

Some people – an alarmingly increasing number influenced by digital 'likes' – seek to preserve the face they had when they were twenty, while others shape their faces to reflect fashion. There are generational, gender, racial and ethnic differences at work. Some people emulate the faces of film stars through plastic surgery, lighting, or cosmetics; a far smaller number use cosmetic surgery to create radically new versions of themselves as tigers or zebras.

Humans are meaning-making creatures, and the stories we tell about ourselves and the world come back, repeatedly, to the face as a symbol and object of power, authenticity, truth and humanity. Why else would each society, across time and place, depict the human face? From cave-wall etchings to the most detailed Renaissance portrait, to the endless proliferation of selfies in the age of Instagram, the face has been imagined, portrayed and commented on – though, critically, in different ways.

What do those portrayals mean? How have they changed? Whose face is being portrayed – and how, and why? This book attempts to answer these questions to reveal the values we place on the face and the person, now and in the past.

As important as representing the face are the ways we know, control, judge and interpret it. Capturing our image matters to our social and familial connections and to our medical, legal and social systems. Today, in our busy, urban landscapes, and our online villages, most of us see more people every day than our ancestors saw in a year – but how many of them can we remember?

Some are more memorable than others, even if you don't have prosopagnosia. And some more beautiful; we like to imagine we can be beautiful too. That quest can become an obsession, as our self-esteem gets bound up in how we look. And no wonder, given the values placed on appearance.

Putting our best face forward is a social as well as a psychological obligation, and we are surrounded by material objects to make that easy; to help us study, change, improve, enhance or despair of our faces – from make-up to injections to implants.

Long before Charlie Brooker's satirical TV series, the 'black mirror' of the ancients, made from obsidian, allowed the wealthy to scrutinize and transform themselves. Today, desire has been democratized, and social media holds up a mirror that reflects and distorts reality. We can change our faces infinitely to suit both our perceived needs and society's expectations: the face has become a commodity we can enhance and improve, in the elusive pursuit of happiness.

We can also, as a last resort, acquire someone else's. Face transplants are a logical extension of our commodification of the body. Just as it has been possible to imagine the body as a machine since the seventeenth century, with the separation of mind and body, we can see ourselves as a series of spare parts. Actual organ donation has only been possible since the 1950s, but now virtually every part of our selves can be replaced.

Things aren't straightforward, though, when it comes to transplanting faces. Given all the meanings the face has been invested with, in areas as diverse as heredity, identity, feeling, beauty, moral and social – even spiritual – worth, how can we replace it with another? And what are the consequences? That's where things get interesting – and controversial.

As the following chapters show, the history of portraying and capturing the face, of reading and interpreting the face, of understanding how we look at faces, and why we try to change and improve them, brings us to the ragged heart of being human. It also points us in the direction of the phenomenon I call facehood: the idea that a single, unique face equates with an individual, named person. Facehood tells us that the possession of a face is a fundamental part of what makes us a unique and indivisible person.

When faces are so invested with psychological and social meanings about our identity and feelings and values, how can we reduce them to commodities, which we hone and shape in the pursuit of

Introduction

happiness? And more fundamentally: can a face transplant be compatible with the values contained in facehood? Spoiler: it can't. And that has profound and challenging consequences.

The face exists as a physical fact and an idealized image, a marker of identity and a product of consumption, a promise of authenticity and a mediator of trust. But the face can also be altered, fabricated and hidden. This ambivalence is why there have been such debates over whether it is socially – even legally – acceptable to cover the face with a mask or an Islamic head covering. Although this book is principally about the West, what we hide and what we reveal of the face, and how that impacts our social relationships, matters to us all.

Let's start our journey with painted faces – exploring how Renaissance portraiture first made faces into markers of individual identity. We'll see how photography democratized faces but also made them vulnerable to surveillance and control. We'll discover how mirrors taught us to see ourselves as others see us, and how that changed everything about the relationship between faces and selfhood. We'll explore the dark history of how faces became tools for categorizing and ranking human worth, creating hierarchies that persist to this day. We'll examine how we construct faces for the dead, revealing our own biases in the process. And we will see how far the idea of facehood withstands a face transplant.

In researching this book, I have interviewed face-transplant surgeons, immunologists, nurses, ethicists, prosthetists, patients and their families. I have poked around in museum exhibits and lain on an fMRI bed to have my own brain scanned. I have interviewed people with facial difference, and facial paralysis, as well as cosmetic surgeons, neuroscientists, psychologists, robotic engineers, philosophers, writers, artists, computer scientists, facial-recognition specialists and sculptors.

I have dug deep in archives and libraries too, researching the histories of portraiture, cosmetic surgery, photography, anthropology, embryology, museums and material culture, psychology and neuroscience. All these disciplines intersect with the human face in ways we have not fully appreciated – and they all construct stories about the face, and what it means, in history and in the present.

Introduction

What I have discovered challenges assumptions and reveals new insights, such as how facial bias has become endemic in society and judicial systems; why we shouldn't reduce prosopagnosia to brain function; how beauty doesn't make us happier; and why we presume a person's true feelings are etched on their face.

All this matters because faces matter more than ever in the digital world. Appearance anxieties are increasing, with newly coined dysmorphias such as 'Zoom chin' as people spend too long staring at their own online image.

Technologies have always intersected with, and reinforced, facial judgements. In the sixteenth century, when mirrors were rarer, sermons linked vanity to sin. But they also taught that the face revealed the soul; you could tell by a stranger's face if they were evil. Today, evolutionary psychology claims we can judge a stranger's identity, morality and worth from their face, in a tenth of a second.

But there's more to the face than God or evolution. Throughout history, the face has been a canvas for projecting beliefs about beauty, identity and worth.

This book explores that canvas, revealing the beliefs, presumptions and prejudices linked to the face, and the mechanisms by which judging ourselves and others has been normalized. It brings together my unique perspective as an academic who has spent 25 years researching the histories of emotion and the body, and a woman with prosopagnosia who has spent fifty years struggling to map this face onto that person. For me, facehood – that automatic equation we make between a unique face and a named individual – has always been elusive.

What I discovered, in bringing these two worlds together, was a new way of thinking about the face, and its role in emotion, identity and communication. I have shared those discoveries in the following pages, and I hope you'll think differently too. After all, there's a lot at stake.

I.

Portrayed

Most children, by the age of three, are masters at drawing faces. At the age of two they might have learned to hold a crayon, with which they scribble ferociously across a page to capture something unguessable to most adults. But by three their focus becomes more intense and predictable, as do the faces that they draw: round heads, raisin eyes and a beaming smile.

This interest in faces is unsurprising; children are reliant on other people for survival, intuitively they know this depends on the social world and their place in it. The more children learn, the more sophisticated their drawings; heads that might once have sprouted arms become heads sitting atop triangular or circular bodies. Faces do not only smile but frown in anger and cry large tears that puddle on the ground. Faces are related to other faces – most often siblings, friends and animals – and to real or imagined places.

Many of us pack up our crayons in secondary school as our creativity becomes something that is judged and graded. But the desire, or need, to portray the human face is untouched. Even if we don't create those images ourselves, we worry about our own faces in the mirror and in photographs, and study voraciously faces presented by others online, in films and on television, in advertising and magazines.

This universal desire, or need, to portray the face does not mean it has always been portrayed in the same way. The faces of the late twentieth-century figurative painter Francis Bacon are markedly different from the 25,000-year-old ivory Venus of Brassempouy (see fig. 1), to Botticelli's fifteenth-century *Birth of Venus*, and to the idealized hyper-realism of Leng Jun's *Mona Lisa – the Design of a Smile*, painted in 2005. These differences are not just about style or ability or materials. They express important attitudes to the idea of the self, and how far the face mirrors the mind.

Can you imagine what it might mean to live in a world where no one remembered your face? Where your individual appearance simply didn't matter? For most people, for thousands of years, this was reality. Today's faces – those that are carefully photographed for Instagram, or scrutinized before an important meeting, or 'touched up' before a date – exist in a completely different cultural context to faces of the past.

For most of human history, portrayals of the face have been generic – more akin thematically to a child's drawing than to post-Renaissance attempts at realism or verisimilitude. Historically, the people represented have not always been specific, named individuals (unless leaders, saints or martyrs). Portrayals of the face were formulaic and symbolic, representing characters and ideals, or social and religious importance, rather than what a person really looked like.

The importance of the face, or at least the head, in saying something about what mattered to human society is evident from the Neolithic skull cults of the Polynesians. But we know that before the Renaissance faces weren't individuated in ways that are important to our modern sense of facehood, that is, a single person being associated with a unique face. This raises a bigger theme that comes up repeatedly in this book: did people look at the face differently in the past? And how far back in history can we go?

Let's take early humans. Experts in human evolution now say that Neanderthals were collaborative and focused on trade as well as creativity. This must have involved more than language, though that is the focus of Yuval Noah Harari's *Sapiens: A Brief History of Humankind* (2011). Human communication relies on body language and facial communication, especially in non-literate societies. It is not easy to study how far the face was important to Neanderthals; we can only get so much information from bone fragments and fossils. What then of the art of early humans?

Although their DNA survives in many of us, Neanderthals died out about 40,000 years ago; some 15,000 years before a Gravettian artist made the Venus of Brassempouy. Early humans also left traces on cave walls and in France; in the Chauvet-Pont-d'Arc Cave, located on a limestone cliff in the Gorges de l'Ardèche. There, archaeologists found stylized depictions of humans and animals – horses, mammoths, bears, leopards, lions and rhinos. We can only guess at the meanings of these figures, but it is notable that human beings are less realistic than the animals depicted.

What does it mean that humans are cyphers in the Chauvet-Pont-d'Arc Cave, or that where humans appear, it is only in relation to animals? Were humans less important? Or were faces simply less important than hands, which are depicted far more often; perhaps not only because daubing a handprint is simpler, but also because hands can hunt and cook and fight?

We find the same lack of attention to human faces in the 17,000-year-old cave paintings in the Lascaux valley. The Hall of Bulls contains 130 figures, 36 of which are equines, stags and bulls. One humanoid has a bird-face, but there is nothing that characterizes a particular individual. However, there is evidence of great artistic skill, and of a kind we normally associate with the Renaissance – the bulls that give the cave its name are drawn with a twisted perspective, their horns front on and their bodies in profile, to give a sense of movement.

It is not a lack of know-how, then, that explains why human faces were absent in Palaeolithic art, or why humans were pictured doing rather than being; hunting, chasing, carrying objects. Speculatively, we might imagine that individual identity was not so important to the structuring of Palaeolithic society as it is today, when faces are everywhere. If people worked collectively and within small groups, and preservation of that connectedness was critical to survival, then perhaps there would be no point in marking out any one individual, or face, as unique. Individualism might even have seemed dangerous.

What of the Venus of Brassempouy (fig. 1), who is usually

The Face

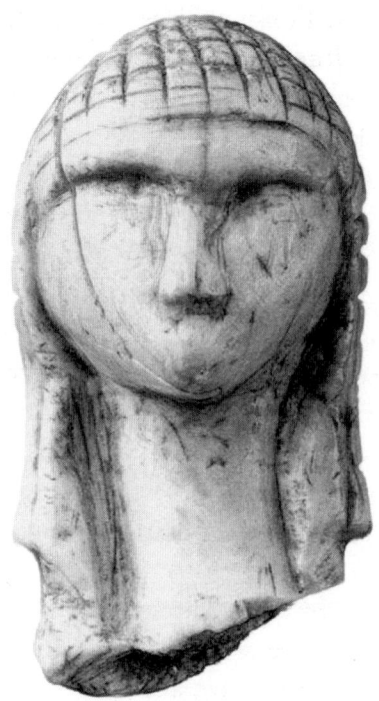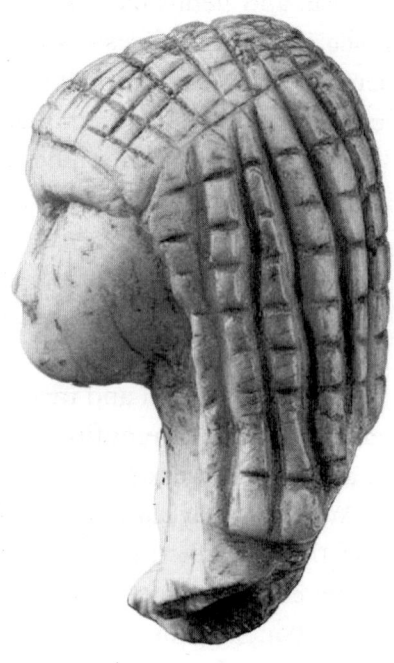

1. The Venus of Brassempouy, c. 25,000 BCE, dating from the Upper Palaeolithic period.

considered to be the earliest representation of a human face? The figure is unsexed, but regarded as female, partly because the cave held broken bodies of other Venuses, with the round hips and breasts that were ancient symbols of fertility. Carved from mammoth tusks, the Venus of Brassempouy has discernible facial features, a forehead, nose and chin, but no mouth. The face is less detailed than the hair or head-covering; indeed, an alternative name for her is 'La Dame à la Capuche' – The Lady with the Hood.

Aegean art was similarly non-committal when it came to facial detail, as we see if we fast-forward several thousand years to 3,000–1,100 BCE. Three distinct civilizations – the Cycladic, Minoan and Mycenaean – lived around the Aegean Sea and the mainland of Greece; their sculpture, especially Cycladic statues, had noses, breasts and Venus-like hips. But they had only rudimentary, symbolic gestures as faces – which later influenced twentieth-century Cubist artists such as Pablo Picasso and Alberto Giacometti, who used geometric shapes to depict people and objects.

By c. 450 BCE something dramatic was changing in how faces were portrayed. The 'Severe' style of sculpture was emerging in Greek art. Most people will know work of this type, since it lines the halls of European collections, including the British Museum and the Acropolis Museum. Attention to the details of the body and the face was more pronounced, with greater interest in characterization, emotion and movement. Limbs showed movement and faces were full of emotion, or intent on managing it, as seen in the marble sculptures of Olympia's Temple of Zeus.

Why did early classical art become so focused on characterization and the face? Picture yourself in Athens during this period – city states constantly at war over land, resources and power; not only Athens and Sparta who fought the Peloponnesian War between 431 and 404 BCE, but also Corinth and Thebes. Even in earlier periods of military tension, a recognizable figurehead was hugely important and artistic style could be as much an identifying feature of a developing society as its political changes: in this case, the emergence of Athenian democracy and, slightly later, the severe style, the hallmark of Greek sculpture in stone and bronze, and in the sculptural decoration of architecture.

There were changes in medicine and science too. Anatomical dissection played a role in artists' interest in the face; understanding how the muscles and nerves of the face worked helped them to capture a person's emotional expressions, even their likeness. There was no formal, recorded dissection until Erasistratus formed an anatomy school in Alexandria, along with fellow physician Herophilus. Then, for a brief time around 300 BCE, there was a close relationship between art and science, and a corresponding interest in realism that would not reappear in the West until Leonardo da Vinci. Even Galen, the Greek physician who in the second century CE famously treated the gladiators of Rome and the emperor

Marcus Aurelius, never dissected a human body. His findings were based on dissections of pigs and monkeys.

In the early classical period, as in the Renaissance, realism was tempered by ideals of beauty. Euclid of Alexandria, who lived around 300 BCE and systematized geometry in his *Elements*, explored what he called 'extreme and mean ratio' – a mathematical proportion later dubbed the 'golden ratio.' This formula for order and perfection (approximately 1:1.618) was believed to exist throughout nature and could be applied to architecture. Also known as the divine proportion, the golden ratio describes how parts of a whole are balanced. In nature that might be the arrangement of petals on a sunflower. Euclid wasn't the first to equate order and harmony with beauty, but many later artists and architects believed this ratio created aesthetically pleasing shapes, influencing Islamic, Buddhist, and Romanesque architecture across centuries.

What does this have to do with faces? Well, the order and proportion of a person's face were similarly judged according to the golden mean. And there were significant implications, since beauty echoed nature and the divine. If the composition of the face reflected the work of God, then it also revealed the state of the soul. 'Only the beautiful were truly good', and 'ill-proportioned men [were] scoundrels' as claimed in *Physiognomics*, a pseudo-Aristotelian work (the term came from Greek physis meaning 'nature' and gnomon meaning 'judge'). Written by followers of Aristotle, who established principles linking physical features to inner nature, it argued a well-proportioned face reflected someone 'just and courageous'.

This belief underpinned another powerful idea that shaped how faces were understood for centuries: that outer appearance – particularly the face – revealed inner character. According to *Physiognomics*, 'brave men had stiff hair, an erect carriage . . . a bright eye', whereas 'the coward had pallor about the face; eyes weak and blinking'. Beauty wasn't just aesthetic – it was moral. The symmetrical, proportional face reflected divine order and a virtuous soul.

The text presumed knowledge of humoral medicine, which dominated the Western tradition from the second to the eighteenth century.

This saw the body as made up of four different humours: phlegm, blood, yellow bile and black bile, the distribution of which determined your personality and what you looked like. A choleric person was physically lean with dry curly hair that was often red; a melancholy person had long hair, since their bodies were wetter and couldn't 'burn up' the excess black bile in their system. Melancholics had pale, moist faces.

Today we might judge by appearances but know that it's unfair. Classical theorists judged by appearances and believed it was essential. When choosing a worker, a friend, a business partner, a lover, it was important to know not only that 'brave men had stiff hair' and 'an erect carriage' and a 'bright eye, neither too wide opened nor half closed' but even more specifically that the forehead is sharp, straight, not large, and lean, neither very smooth nor very wrinkled'. The coward had less blood than the brave man, which gave him 'pallor about the face; eyes weak and blinking . . . the expression on his face is liable to rapid change and is cowed'.

When you read the face in classical Greece, it was important to study humans and animals together. There was overlap between the temperaments of animals and humans, and these could be detected in facial features. As *Physiognomics* continued:

> Those who have thin lips and slack parts at the joining of the lips, so that the upper lip overhangs the lower at the join, are magnanimous; witness the lions. One can see the same thing in large and powerful dogs. Those that have thin hard lips, prominent in the neighbourhood of the canine teeth, such are of noble nature; witness the boar. But those that have thick lips with the upper projecting over the lower are dull; witness asses and monkeys . . . Creatures with a fleshy face are lazy; witness cattle . . . Those with small faces are little-minded; this applies to the cat and the monkey. Those with large faces are sluggish; witness asses and cattle. But since the face should be neither small nor large, the state between these two is the most satisfactory.

Despite his influence, physiognomy wasn't invented by Aristotle; people judged by looks as early as 1500 BCE, as seen in Mesopotamian handbooks on divination. In 500 BCE Pythagoras allegedly accepted students based on their facial appearance. Ancient Egyptians similarly regarded beauty as a sign of holiness, and ancient India's enlightened Siddhars read spirituality in the face.

In the Spring and Autumn periods of Chinese history (c. 770–481 BCE), face-reading revealed a person's character, personality and future. According to the *Book of Rites*, 'those who look up are arrogant; those who look down are worried; those who look sideways are sly'. Face-reading still thrives in traditional Chinese medicine, and as we will see, in modern facial-recognition systems.

This belief that the face revealed character wasn't just artistic theory. It shaped how people judged one another in daily life, and it influenced portrayals of the face – it is one reason why Greek statues have symmetrical, stylized faces.

Precisely because faces were key to a person's social and moral status – as well as cultural identity and communication – facial mutilation, including eye gouging, ear hacking and nose amputation, were routine punishments in classical Greece and the Persian Empire, just as they were in Republican and Imperial Rome. Facial mutilation was also linked to specific criminal offences, especially sexual offences – this would echo the 'God-given' punishment of smallpox or syphilis for sexual promiscuity, diseases and infections that often disfigured the face.

These forms of punishment survived to the Byzantine period and were common in early modern Europe. (Outside of crime and punishment, damaging a woman's face was particularly devastating; today, acid attacks on women are rising as a form of social and 'honour-based' punishment.)

According to the second-century CE Greek geographer Pausanias, Herakles, known to the Romans as Hercules, was named Rhinokoloustes (Nose-docker) because he liked to chop off the noses of heralds. There was even a region on the border of ancient Egypt and Israel called *Rhinocorura*, which means 'cut-off noses' in Greek; it was founded by the Ethiopian king Actisanes as a place of exile for robbers without noses.

Statues of unpopular leaders have always had their faces mutilated too – and not just statues. It's recorded in medieval manuscripts that the nose of the Byzantine emperor Justinian II was chopped off during a revolt. Emperors more than anyone else needed to reflect the perfect image of God; they could not afford to be disfigured. So, after he was deposed, Justinian acquired a gold prosthetic nose, which he wore to enable him to take back the throne.

After Rome conquered Corinth (146 BCE), Roman leaders copied the famous marble and bronze statues of Greek leaders which had been made by artists such as Praxiteles. Most Roman sculptors were not so skilled, but they did introduce verism, which prioritized hyper-realistic and idealized traits. From Augustus, the first emperor, onwards, Roman leaders used statues in propaganda, and in ways that implied a mythological heritage or military lineage.

Unlike Greek portraiture, which celebrated youth, symmetry and firmness, sculptural portraits like Head of a Roman Patrician from Otricoli (fig. 2) conveyed seriousness and intellect through facial wrinkles, which were respected – in men. The Patrician has a stoic expression, and a furrowed brow intended to show depth of thought. Because physical strength symbolized mental strength, it was not unusual for such sculptures to have a bizarre duality: the

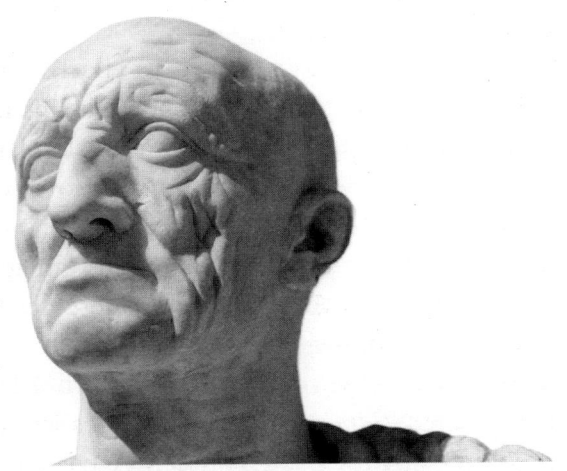

2. Head of a Roman Patrician from Otricoli, c. 75–50 BCE.

taut and muscled body of an athlete rendered in marble, alongside a wizened head and face. The symbolic function – that this was a man of virility, strength and wisdom – mattered more than any actual resemblance.

However, it is likely that Roman portrait statues were more objectively 'realistic' than their predecessors, and this is because wax masks were used to capture the image of an individual while living or dead. The right to do this, and to have an imago of oneself to keep for posterity, was exclusive to aristocrats, those who held the highest positions of power in the Republic. Family members might even wear the masks at funerals to honour the person who had died. After death, these masks were passed down through the family as evidence of their pedigree.

Why did Roman private portraiture flourish? The main reason was the symbolic and literal importance of the figurehead. For politicians, athletes, gods, demigods, philosophers, orators and poets – and to a far lesser degree noblewomen and even children, though of course this too reflected glory on the husband and father – there was no greater sign of respect than the honorific sculpture. Female faces were not subjected to the verism found in male portraiture: they remained relatively generic and idealized. Passive beauty rather than active presence was expected from wives and mothers.

The general move towards recognizability makes sense when we consider the increasingly common use of a ruler's face on legal currency. Not all leaders are easily recognizable, and in any case, very few ordinary people saw them in person. In hierarchical and pre-literate societies, symbols have always stood in for recognizability. Macedonian coinage adapted Greek symbols to emphasize stability and continuity in leadership. On a tetradrachm, a silver coin worth four drachmae, the head of Alexander the Great is shown as conqueror of India. He wears an elephant scalp with tusks, and a craning trunk. Pictured on the reverse is Zeus, the father of the gods. It is not clear whether this coin, or the series, the 'elephant coinage', was struck during Alexander's lifetime. The face hints at a living and distinct person, with a straight nose, a slightly protruding jaw, a pronounced forehead and deep-set eyes. But as important, it was a symbol of power carrying on after his death.

Alexander would have known the impact of physiognomic beliefs; when he was thirteen years old, his tutor for ethics and politics was Aristotle. And so, on coinage, Alexander's strong chin signalled masculine virtues of strength and courage; his wide eyes indicated vision and intelligence, his full lips represent generosity and eloquence, and his large eyes showed he was not 'little-minded', nor anything like a monkey.

Pagan statues from the second and first centuries BCE were defaced, as Emperor Constantine adopted Christianity as his favoured cult. It wasn't novel for sculpture to be created and destroyed and repurposed, but crosses being carved into the faces of pagan gods was something new: a graphic act of appropriation, about who and what should be worshipped. This gesture also powerfully rejected the individual face as important – especially the female faces of ancient goddesses. Many works of art were destroyed. By the fifth century CE, skilled sculptors and their materials were harder to find in the West. And so, any new sculpture created across the Roman Empire tended to be architectural and Christian.

Portraiture took time, skill and money. So, it's no surprise that historically it has been linked to the wealthy. The idea that a commoner would have their image captured for posterity was unthinkable; there would be no purpose, and no resources to make it possible. Who would pay to commemorate the face of a peasant? And why would one peasant need to be differentiated from another in the absence of power or wealth, or leadership or bureaucratic systems, or any reason to preserve individual likeness? The lack of need, opportunity and purpose meant that portraiture would not be democratized for centuries. It would, however, become more individuated.

I should add that there are occasional examples of individuation in early portraiture. Among the best known are the Fayum mummy portraits of second-century CE Egypt (fig. 3); a series of naturalistic painted portraits on wooden boards. After the combined forces of

The Face

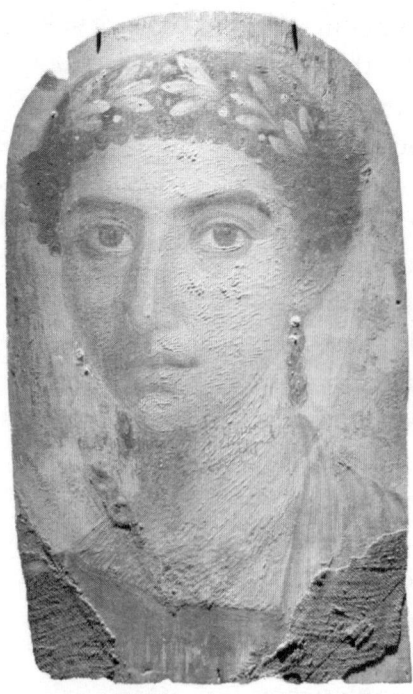

3. Mummy portrait of Eirene, 50 CE.

Antony and Cleopatra lost the Battle of Actium in 31 BCE, Egypt became part of the Roman Empire a year later, and these kinds of realistic paintings became a new trend for burials. The Fayum portraits came from respected Greco-Roman families, and we can imagine that they were carrying on the tradition of imago by other means. It is also likely that, as with the wax masks made for the Roman elite, these wooden-boarded portraits were created during a person's life and intended to celebrate family status as much as that person's uniqueness.

What was happening outside of Europe? Although this book focuses on Western history, and portraiture was largely a Western tradition that developed alongside individualistic philosophy, China had a history of interest in the face. As in the West, that interest was principally about godly beings (ancestors), or stylized leaders, and human figures were largely undifferentiated. Early Chinese art showed human beings in relation to a set of signs of activity. Human figurines in the fourth century BCE focused on people doing rather than being: a man with a lamp, a servant carrying a tray, with faces that were homogeneous and typified. Similarly, Persian portraiture, which borrowed from the artistic traditions of Assyria, Egypt and Mycenae, mostly focused on male, royal figures, and even the regal reliefs on tombs did not attempt to capture the facial likeness of the dead. As in China, motifs from plants and nature and animals took priority, along with scenes of faceless workers.

Some religious cultures, including the Judaic and Islamic traditions, had a prohibition on idolatry and 'graven images' that included the face. Although Shia Islam is more tolerant of images of human figures, Islamic tradition generally prohibits all images of Muhammed and defamatory images are especially offensive. Which is why the 2007 Swedish cartoon by Lars Vilks that depicted the prophet's head on a dog's body caused such controversy. The cartoon also represented an inversion of an ancient tradition – cynocephaly, the mythological depiction of human figures with dog heads found in Egypt, India, Greece and China. The Egyptian god Anubis is an example most readers will know. By reversing this (and placing a man's head on a dog's body), the cartoon subverted millennia of how the human-animal appearance boundary has been represented in art.

What happened to faces after the fall of the Western Roman Empire in the fifth century might surprise you. In the Christian tradition, there had been no barrier to representing the faces of humans, but the face was less significant in medieval art than in the classical period. Why? It wasn't about skill, though the 'Dark Ages' have been wrongly labelled as lacking in it. There was plenty of artistic ability about, as evidenced by the great cathedrals filled with sculpture, paintings and stained glass. So how do we account for the decline in facial portraiture?

There are a few possible explanations for this shift. After the fall of the Western Roman Empire, medieval Europe divided into smaller kingdoms and feudal territories; power was more diffuse, and traditions varied. What was universal was the rise of Christianity as a dominant Western religion from the early fourth century under Emperor Constantine, which brought about a focus on the celebration of the divine – especially in illuminated manuscripts and Gothic cathedrals – rather than honouring specific human individuals. When specific individuals *were* portrayed, it tended to be within stylized religious contexts – one example is the first Holy Roman Emperor, Charlemagne, who appeared in several important Carolingian manuscripts, most notably the Vienna Coronation Gospels (c. 795 CE), to show that his authority was divine.

With Christianity came religious sensibilities about the body and resurrection that made anatomical dissection uncommon and controversial until the thirteenth century and the Renaissance anatomical revolution. In the fourteenth and fifteenth centuries, dissections were mainly for teaching, and mostly confined to medical schools and universities. Even within these parameters dissections were viewed with suspicion by religious authorities, and there were social restrictions – dissection tended to be limited to the executed bodies of criminals. In England in the 1500s, the Company of Barber-Surgeons, later known as the Royal College of Surgeons, permitted only four executed criminals to be dissected annually for teaching. In Italy, artists gained greater access through established medical schools. By the late fifteenth century, Leonardo da Vinci in Florence and Milan obtained regular access to cadavers for systematic study, making it possible for artists to understand the underlying structure of the face and facial expressions.

(There would still, however, be a scarcity of bodies for dissection until the Victorian period, which explains the lucrative but scandalous 'grave-robbing' of William Burke and William Hare; the term is a misnomer, for they were murderers who sold the corpses of their victims for the purposes of dissection in anatomy lectures.)

What might it have been like to live during this time, of limited anatomical knowledge and religious constraints on representation; without mirrors, photographs and personal portraits? You'd have only the vaguest notion of your own appearance. Your identity would be defined by your role, your family, your village and your faith – not by your individual face. The idea that your specific features mattered enough that you should preserve and even enhance them would have seemed strange, perhaps even verging dangerously on pride.

You would, however, know well the faces of the people you were answerable to, who would probably be members of the same family that dated back several generations. Unlike anonymous urban populations, rural dwellers had less need to read a person's face to determine their character – so physiognomy mattered less. It was still taught at European universities as part of natural philosophy, and used in literature to help detect strangers, as in 'The Tale of Beryn', a spurious addition to Chaucer's *The Canterbury Tales*: 'I knowe wele by thy fisnamy, thy kynd were to stele.' But the decline in literacy and knowledge of Latin also meant reduced access to the texts that had reinforced Greco-Roman ideas, and physiognomic principles were bastardized or used satirically, as they were in *The Canterbury Tales*; 'the Pardoner' had bulging eyes and a high-pitched voice, both characteristics associated with effeminacy and shamelessness, though the character was supposed to embody religious virtue. Finally, the development of medieval artistic traditions, with bright colours, jewels and Christian symbolism, conveyed a world seen through splendour and faith, not through the study of individual faces.

Medieval portraiture did continue throughout Europe, but early medieval England lacked the rich tradition of royal commemoration existing in Byzantine Greek, Ottonian German and Carolingian Frankish courts. English images of kings focused on heraldry or religious symbolism to show who a leader was; one well-known example is the Wilton Diptych, made for Richard II. Coinage still carried the image of rulers, and there was more focus on royal portraiture in England with the arrival of the Normans and the Plantagenets. From the fourteenth century onward, portraits of English monarchs became more standardized: iconic images of Henry V and Richard III in the fifteenth century display the visual propaganda we now associate with early modern monarchies, by the time nation states began to separate from the Roman Catholic Church.

The Face

Outside the royal courts, and across Europe, monks who created illuminated manuscripts were only interested in individual faces if they belonged to saints or donors. Medieval portraiture was valued for its ability to express a person's social status, religious convictions or political position. Monarchs were given more distinctive facial appearances, since they needed to be recognizable, but otherwise artists focused on the clothing, heraldry or objects that gave a person their social value.

The rarity of paintings helps explain this approach. Formal portraits were few and far between and were intended to show a person how they wished to be remembered over multiple generations. This is very different from our 'selfie' culture in which images are easy to produce, reproduce and disseminate. We might capture a moment, but seldom for posterity. Christ and the saints needed to be recognizable instantly, to many people and over a long period. This could only be achieved by the artist's skills in symbolism, positioning, clothing and gestures.

Consider a medieval illumination of *Saint Hedwig of Silesia* (fig. 4). In this image, the saint carries an ivory statue of the Madonna and Child, and a little prayer book. A pair of long, soft boots are draped over her arm, symbolizing that Hedwig went barefoot in imitation of the Apostles, but her lace-trimmed robe reminds viewers she was also a member of the aristocracy before she entered a nunnery. The manuscript's patrons, descendants of Hedwig, kneel before her on either side. It was the social positioning of Hedwig via these artefacts that made her identifiable to illiterate subjects, rather than her face. Personal identity came second to social and religious position.

Outside the courts and the Church, faces were everywhere, though rarely depicted with realism. While paintings immortalized biblical figures and tales, and sculpted heads of nobles were used to show power and leadership, stone faces in cathedrals and churches were cartoonish. In and on Romanesque and Gothic churches, medieval faces stuck out their tongues, gnashed their teeth, rolled their eyes and roared in anger. Gargoyles – the word derives from the Latin *gurgulio*, *gula*, *gargula* (gullet or throat) – served a practical

Portrayed

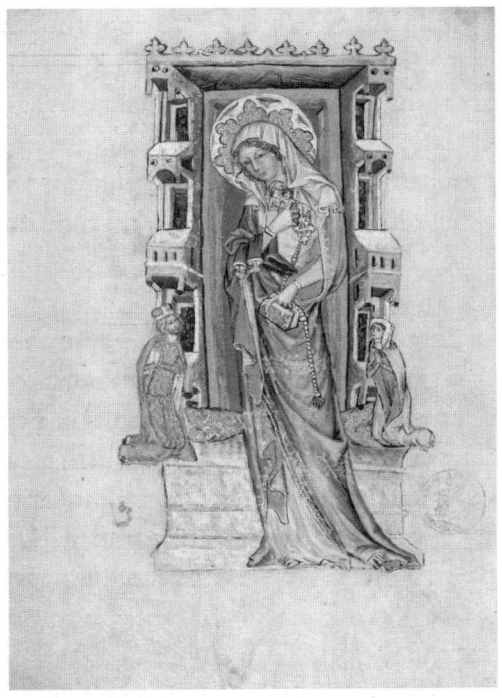

4. Nicolaus of Prussia, *Saint Hedwig of Silesia*, 1353.

function in transporting water from roofs, but they were also symbolic in protecting against evil, or warning of the perils of hell for the impious.

Anthropomorphic faces, lions most often, might have helped convert pagans by appropriating familiar imagery. Gargoyles that were bawdy and comedic had a social as well as political function by representing the sins of the prostitute, the drunk or the moneylender. Corbel heads, stone or wood images of faces, were more realistic and represented generic people, though sometimes in mocking ways; it wasn't unusual for corbels to be hidden in the eaves of churches, where stonemasons could send secret messages of contempt toward those they despised – rival architects, overbearing priests, or perhaps even the master mason.

The extreme emotions displayed on gargoyles and corbels also portrayed the foolishness of human passions as compared to the calm, measured face of Christ. The conventional image of a bearded Jesus with long hair emerged in the first century, but it didn't become common until the sixth century in Eastern Christianity, and much later in the West. Some medieval Western images of Jesus' face, usually of the 'Meeting at Emmaus', where his disciples didn't recognize their master after his resurrection, show Jesus wearing a Jewish hat.

But Christ's appearance in art is most associated with calm resignation – turning the other cheek – to show that outward displays of emotion were sinful and rebellious. An important exception to this image of Jesus were depictions of him in pain during his crucifixion, which were prominent in late medieval art, especially the Gothic period. Artists aimed to evoke strong emotional responses from viewers by portraying the physical suffering of Christ; the trend continued into the Renaissance, when a more expansive understanding of the emotions emerged in art.

Then came an explosion of interest in the individual human face that still shapes our world today. What happened?

As a woolworker in fifteenth-century Florence, you would likely be unaware of the dramatic cultural changes that we now know as the Renaissance. Your world would consist of your family, your neighbourhood, your trade and your parish church; you might notice more construction projects as wealthy families commissioned impressive buildings and artworks, but the grand intellectual and artistic movements taking shape in the palaces and studios of the wealthy would have been unknown to you, quite separate from your world of wool dust and aching backs.

In historical retrospect, however, trade during the Renaissance was booming, the Gutenberg printing press was spreading new ideas – not only in Latin, but also in German, French and English. Ancient Greek and Roman texts were being rediscovered and artists like Leonardo da Vinci were dissecting corpses to understand the underlying structures of the human body as they sought to create ever more realistic artworks.

It is no coincidence that the fifteenth century also saw the professionalization of European portrait painting. Humanism, which originated in northern Italy in the late thirteenth and fourteenth centuries, promoted the idea that Man was the centre of the universe, and human achievements could celebrate humanity as well as God.

The developments in international trade and finance during the Renaissance also opened new lands to new peoples; a market for art and self-promotion developed at the same time as artists began to be celebrated for their individual genius. They were exemplars of humanism, after all. New ways of thinking about the world, from the rebirth of the golden ratio, to shifts in astronomy, mathematics, medicine and science, suggested that the possibilities for the individual were endless. As Shakespeare's Hamlet (1599-1601) declared: 'What a piece of work is man! How noble in reason! How infinite in faculty! In form and moving how express and admirable! In action how like an angel! In apprehension how like a god!'

Even now the Western world remains significantly in thrall to the Renaissance, and to the belief that our individuality and feelings matter. The Renaissance is seen as one of the most important artistic periods in history: perhaps it is taught so often in schools because Renaissance portraits and self-portraits are recognizably 'modern' in their emotions and facial expressions. The men and women depicted certainly feel, and look, more 'like us' than their severely styled forebears, or Greco-Roman statues.

Consider Hans Holbein the Younger's 1527 *Portrait of Sir Thomas More*, from one of the most celebrated artists of the sixteenth century (fig. 5). This is one of twenty-three portraits of More, though he may have sat for more than that. Holbein painted him dressed in the livery chain of office with Tudor rose, which is a sign of fealty and high office, and a fur-lined coat of black satin and red velvet, a colour and material that the sumptuary laws restricted to the elite. (Henry VIII ensured that nobody below the rank of knight could wear velvet or crimson; only royals could wear gold, and Henry routinely wore red and gold.)

More's portrait includes a cord at the upper right that is tied in

The Face

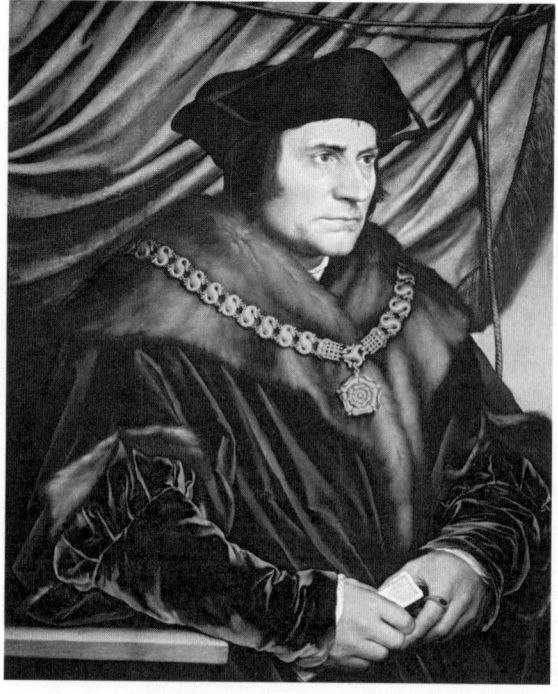

5. Sir Thomas More (1478–1535) portrait painting by Hans Holbein the Younger, 1527.

a loose Franciscan knot, a sign of his spiritual convictions, and he is holding a book, which symbolizes knowledge. All these symbols would have communicated More's status and power to anyone fortunate enough to view the picture hanging in a palace, château or private home. Importantly, the portrait also gives a clear sense of a psychologically strong and resolute human being: his chin is lifted, and his eyes are fixed straight ahead, as though fixated on something beyond human concerns. We may be more inclined to see this because we know More was executed by Henry VIII for his refusal to acknowledge him as the Head of the Church of England. But even allowing for that retrospective judgement, Holbein evidently wanted to capture a specific and important person, not just a figurehead.

Why was this shift towards individualized portraiture so significant?

Up to this point in history, to be portrayed at all was a privilege reserved for the powerful. Now, for the first time, we see artists taking an interest in capturing not just status but personality – that ineffable quality that makes each human unique. The face had begun its journey from being a symbol of power or piety to being a window into the individual soul.

Holbein's work was influenced by another great artist, Leonardo da Vinci – Indeed, Holbein's *The Last Supper* (1524–5) was inspired by Leonardo's painting of the same name, and Leonardo's anatomical dissections informed his analysis of the human face. His *Mona Lisa* (fig. 6) is probably the most famous portrait in the world. Painted in oils on poplar wood, it is thought to show a Florentine noblewoman called Lisa del Giocondo – hence the portrait's other name: '*La Gioconda*'. She was not from an especially important family, but artists needed to make a living, and Leonardo was probably between commissions.

What makes this portrait revolutionary isn't its subject, but its execution. Through techniques like *sfumato* (subtle blending around

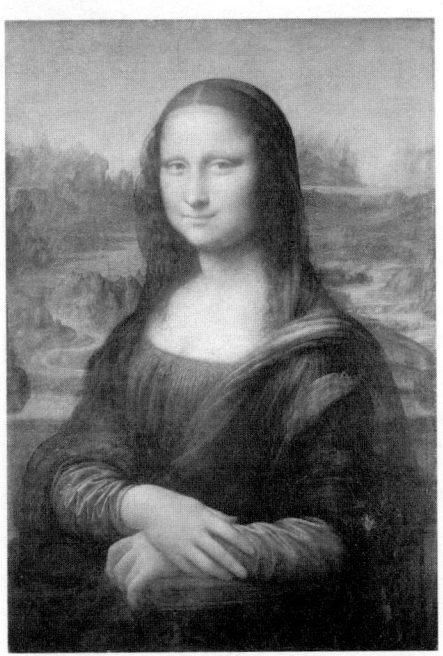

6. Leonardo da Vinci, *Mona Lisa*, c. 1503–19.

the eyes and mouth), Leonardo created a softness of expression that suggests interior thoughts and emotions. The eyes of the sitter meet those of the viewer and appear to follow them around the room. And that enigmatic smile suggests an emotional ambiguity that had never before been captured in portraiture.

Stylistically, the painting follows the conventions required for fifteenth- and sixteenth-century virtuous womanhood: the sitter is seated and turned partly towards the viewer; her dark, shoulder-length hair is covered by a translucent veil. She is wearing a modest dark dress, and no jewels. Her right hand is placed over her left in a gesture of faithful wifeliness. With her relatively broad forehead and dark eyes, the overall look is one of Spanish-influenced high fashion; this might have been a step up from how the sitter appeared in everyday life (not all nobles were wealthy), and we do not know the circumstances of the commission with any certainty – but this was presumably how she wanted to be seen.

The completion of the painting was delayed, however, because Leonardo accepted another commission. When he died, his apprentice, then assistant (and some historians have argued his lover), Salai, inherited the painting, and he sold it to King Francis I of France. It has been on display in the Louvre since 1797, where it receives around six million visitors a year, drawn as much by its fame as by its artistic value.

What is it about this portrait that makes it so popular? Most visitors are startled by how small it is, measuring just 77 cm by 53 cm, which was average by Renaissance standards. Only the very wealthy could afford life-size or even larger portraits; even Holbein's portrait of Sir Thomas More was just 74 cm by 59 cm. Compare that to the larger-than-life *Portrait of Henry VIII*, painted by Holbein, which would have adorned the king's privy chamber at Westminster, and stands at 2.5 m by 1.3 m.

The size of a painting influenced its cost to the sitter because it involved more of the artist's time and their materials. To understand why portraits were so prestigious and associated with the rich, we must remember that having a portrait painted would cost the equivalent of a year's wages for a skilled worker. If you wanted to be painted by Holbein or Leonardo, the cost might be equivalent to a property purchase.

Was the *Mona Lisa* worth the cost? Not to the sitter, perhaps, who never actually acquired it. But to others, most notably the Italian painter Giorgio Vasari, best known for writing *Lives of the Artists*, 'all who saw it thought it was wonderful and as real as life itself'.

Since we do not know what the sitter looked like, we cannot tell how faithful the likeness was; Leonardo arguably used the divine proportion beloved by classical artists to achieve order and proportion. If we look at the painting as a series of rectangles, we find that the width of the sitter's forehead is a perfect ratio for the length of her face, as is the proportion of her head length compared to the width of her eyes, and so on.

Today, it is the twentieth-century fame of the painting – helped by its well-publicized theft in 1911 by a former employee at the Louvre – rather than any inherent (yet indisputable) artistic quality, that gives the *Mona Lisa* such widespread popular appeal. Of course, people flock to interpret that famous enigmatic smile for themselves. But the drive towards realism was significant for its time, and something that artists following Leonardo were keen to achieve. Don't forget that he spent some time dissecting corpses to understand the inner workings of the human anatomy, so that he could create the most realistic faces and bodies imaginable. Most other artists did not have the time, the skill or the expertise.

Since it was dull and time-consuming to sit still for a portrait, and many sitters were busy people with many social engagements, artists drew or painted their own faces in the pursuit of realism. The German artist Albrecht Dürer created a series of self-portraits from the age of thirteen. He portrayed himself in various poses, in profile, full-frontal, in costumes, pointing out where his stomach hurt, naked, and even as a provocative rendering of Christ, *Self-Portrait at Twenty-Eight* (fig. 7). Each self-portrait was intended perhaps for a different recipient (art historians have suggested they were gifts to a fiancée, a physician, a patron). The element of performance is important, as is the sense that the artist is present as a distinct person with a recognizable face.

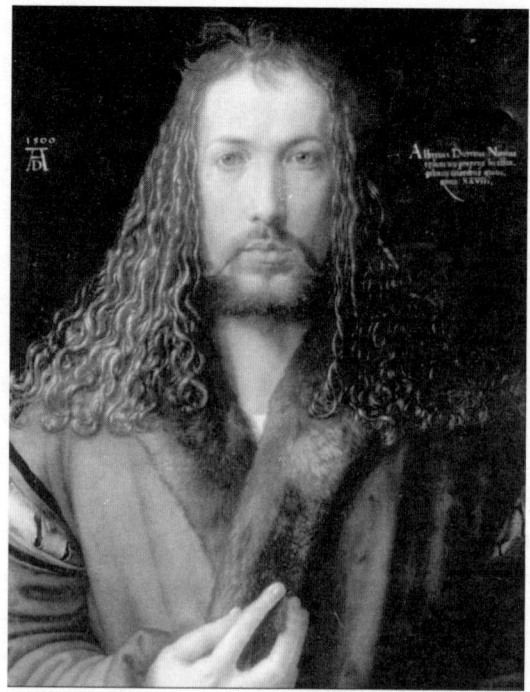

7. Albrecht Dürer, *Self-Portrait at Twenty-Eight*, 1500.

Reusing faces was a common trick in portraiture, and artists often appeared in their own work as bystanders or subjects. Caravaggio painted himself into many portraits, most often as Bacchus, the Roman god of wine; Vermeer painted himself in two of his works, *The Procuress* (as the smiling cavalier) and *The Art of Painting* (the painter with his back to us). *Still Life with Cheeses, Almonds and Pretzels* by the seventeenth-century Flemish artist Clara Peeters contains a reflection of the artist's face, peeking out from a pewter lid.

How did Dürer, and other artists who painted themselves into portraits, know their own faces so well? Well, mirrors were becoming more available. Their improved quality allowed a heightened sense of realism, particularly in skin tone and texture, that was characteristic of Renaissance paintings.

And that's not all. Artistic conventions now focused more on hints of the sitter's inner psychology or state of mind, personality, and even relationship to the artist. In Rembrandt's portrait of the cabinet-maker Herman Doomer, there is a smiling ease to the sitter, as though he feels comfortable in the company of the artist. As it happens, Rembrandt also painted a companion piece of Doomer's wife, Baertje, and the couple's son Lambert was an apprentice in Rembrandt's studio.

Studying faces in the ways that portrait artists did meant that they had to pay close attention to human emotions. If you imagine the face of a loved one, it is probably animated in ways that give them personality: a smile, a frown, a perplexed expression. Starting with the Renaissance, 'the passions' were not ridiculed as they were in medieval gargoyles or looked down on as they had been by Christian or Greco-Roman stoics. Rather they were celebrated as God-given – depending on what the emotions were, and who was expressing them. In this period, the emotions of women, slaves or peasants were not considered a suitable subject for painters, whereas the emotions of important men, the wealthy, the saintly or martyred (men and women) were. Moreover, jealousy and rage were not depicted nearly to the same extent as the emotions of love and compassion.

Building on the anatomical details depicted by Leonardo and Andreas Vesalius, an anatomist and physician who in 1543 published the first anatomical atlas, *On the Fabric of the Human Body in Seven Books*, artists became absorbed by depicting realistic facial expressions. The French painter Charles Le Brun, a founding member in 1648 of the Royal Academy of Painting and Sculpture in Paris, set out important rules for how artists should depict each emotion – which we will explore in detail in a later chapter.

Le Brun's description of emotions like anger, which reddened the face and furrowed the brow, became useful not only for painters, but also actors, and in later centuries for psychologists and criminologists. Understanding and labelling the expressions of the face invited viewers to make an emotional connection and understand what was being portrayed. It was part of the process by which a name was put to a face, rather than to a crown or a story or a virtue.

Beyond the painters' intentions, what did sitters want from a portrait? Rulers wanted to show who ruled, others to show who they were, and what they had achieved. We can imagine most people also wanted to be flattered. Not so, Oliver Cromwell, Roundhead leader during the English Civil War, later Lord Protector. Unlike Charles I and the other royals painted by the Dutch artist Peter Lely, Cromwell famously demanded that he be painted 'truly like me . . . pimples, warts and everything as you see me', giving rise to our well-known expression, 'warts and all'.

As it happens, Royalist writers did not mock Cromwell's warts, which are visible in his death mask, but they did make fun of his large, bulbous, red nose, which suggested drunkenness and syphilis. Even without reference to that nose, Lely produced a portrait that was less flattering and 'royal' than his previous ones. Given his roots as a Puritan, Cromwell dressed simply and there is little ornamentation in the portrait to distract the viewer's eye from the sitter's gaze.

After the Restoration, Lely went back to painting royalty, while Cromwell's body was exhumed from Westminster Abbey and his head put on a long pole affixed to the roof of Westminster Hall. What better way to display the vanity of ambition, and the rottenness of a jumped-up head of state, than by placing his decaying face on a pole?

Lely's other portraits are very different from his painting of Cromwell. For example, *Elizabeth Murray, Lady Tollemache, later Countess of Dysart and Duchess of Lauderdale (1626–1698) and an Unidentified Attendant* (c. 1651) relies on the symbols and finery that traditionally surround portrayals of the wealthy, including the crouching figure of a Black person to reflect the transatlantic slaving interests of the duchess's family.

Most of the portraits discussed so far are of white faces – reflecting centuries of hierarchy and power. It was fashionable from the seventeenth century for Black servants in aristocratic homes to be included in portraits, as a reference to wealth, status and exoticism. Sometimes described as slave-servants (slavery had no formal legal basis in the U.K.), they were often of indeterminate status.

Black servants in aristocratic paintings are posed to the side, turned away, in shadow, or crouched, their faces looking up at the main sitter with a supplicatory expression.

Black faces were seldom given any detail or individuality, just wide eyes with the whites showing against the darkness of their skin and the background of the painting as they handed some exotic offering, an orange perhaps, to the sitter. Sometimes Black servants were dressed in a collar, or a white hand was placed on their head to indicate their subordinate status.

There were important exceptions. In 1649, Juan de Pareja was a slave in the studio of the Spanish artist Velázquez (fig. 8). Enslaved labour was common in the Spanish studios of painters, silversmiths, sculptors and woodworkers. The Spanish guild regulations banned Velázquez from teaching his trade to an enslaved artisan, but Pareja would have carried out basic tasks, such as stretching canvases and

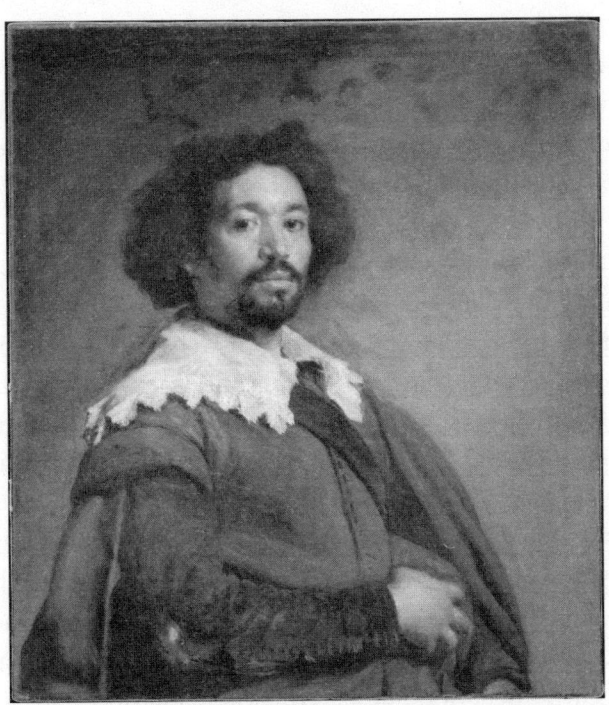

8. Diego Rodríguez de Silva y Velázquez, *Juan de Pareja*, c. 1650.

grinding pigments. He was enslaved by Velázquez for two decades, and yet in his portrait, Pareja looks out at the viewer with his head held high. Soon after the portrait was exhibited, to much critical acclaim for the artist, Velázquez set Pareja free. Pareja went on to become a successful artist in his own right.

Black people were occasionally depicted as free citizens before the abolition of slavery in 1865 by the United States – though transatlantic voyages continued until 1873. The writer and abolitionist Olaudah Equiano (also known as Gustavus Vassa) was painted for a frontispiece to his 1789 autobiography, *The Interesting Narrative of the Life of Olaudah Equiano*. That memoir recounted how Equiano had been captured in present-day Nigeria, shipped to the Caribbean, and sold as a slave to a Royal Navy officer before he bought his freedom in 1766. There is no supplication in Equiano's face or posture. Dressed as a refined, learned gentleman, with the high forehead that was European shorthand for intelligence and civility, Equiano stares back at the viewer, just as Pareja had done.

Because portraits communicated a story to viewers, not only about a person's looks, but also about their status, temperament and role in the world, they were also used in brokering marriage. In the fifteenth century, Jan van Eyck was sent to make portraits of potential wives for his patron, Philip the Good of Burgundy. And who can forget poor Anne of Cleves, Henry VIII's fourth wife? Henry had married Anne in 1540; they met only after the king had sent his court artist, Hans Holbein, to Cleves in the northern Rhineland to paint her portrait. Henry was pleased enough when he saw it but not when Anne arrived in court; it was not a likeness, claimed the disgruntled king. There is no evidence that Henry himself used the words 'Flanders Mare' to describe Anne, but he clearly found her unattractive. Unconsummated, the marriage was annulled in the same year.

By the seventeenth century, miniatures were routinely shared by courting couples and spouses, who wanted to keep their loved ones close. Wealthy merchants commissioned larger-scale portraits too, especially in the Netherlands, then a world power. Frans Hals's

The Laughing Cavalier (fig. 9), a name given by the Victorians to one of the most well-known Dutch portraits of the age, was probably intended as a betrothal portrait. Its subject is neither laughing nor a cavalier, but likely a wealthy cloth merchant – and probably Tieleman Roosterman, a Dutchman who was the subject of another portrait by Hals.

It is the upturned moustache that gives the sense of a smile, so important in capturing the essence of a personality, and the man's jacket is embroidered with motifs of love, including arrows and lovers' knots. The sitter has a half-smile, a twinkling in the eye, and a swaggering pose; whoever this man was, he looked happy with his lot.

What a move away from medieval portraiture, when paintings were intended to depict status and power or piety, rather than individual character! By the seventeenth century, artists no longer

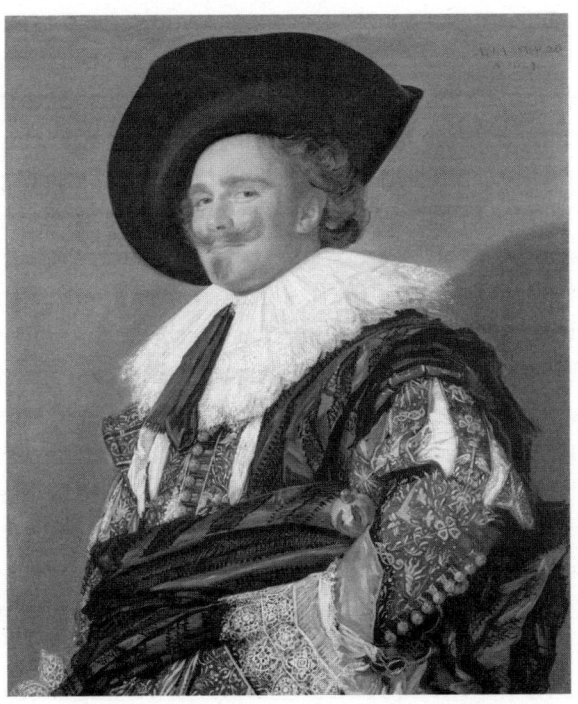

9. Frans Hals, *The Laughing Cavalier*, 1624.

worked primarily for the Church, royalty or rich nobility, as the middle class made wealthy through trade became the most important patrons. This changed the nature of artistic production, as rather than waiting to be commissioned, individual painters could offer their services to prospective buyers. Some artists specialized in portraits, others in landscapes, or history painting, which included a revived interest in allegory and mythological images.

This return to allegory and myth is important, because as we have seen the face has always been shorthand for communicating a person's values. Artists during the Enlightenment loved allegory, and they revisited classical art by dressing up wealthy women as ancient goddesses, shorthand for grace, beauty and goodness. Given the simultaneous revival of an interest in physiognomy, sitters had to be shown as beautiful both inside and out. Portraits again acquired the decorative elements of classical mythology – laurel wreaths, rosettes and acanthus leaves – while the human figure and face were idealized like sculpture.

These changing patterns of patronage and subject matter gave rise to two major artistic movements. The Baroque style, which dominated European art from the early seventeenth century, embraced drama, movement and emotional intensity to serve both the Counter-Reformation's religious aims and the grandeur of absolute monarchs like Louis XIV. Baroque artists such as Caravaggio, Bernini and Rubens created works that were theatrical and dynamic, with faces that displayed intense emotions and psychological depth – a new kind of realism that made religious and mythological figures appear vividly human and immediate.

By the early eighteenth century, as court life became more intimate and refined, the Baroque evolved into the lighter, more decorative Rococo style. Rococo artists like Watteau, Boucher and Fragonard favoured pastel colours, playful themes and ornate decoration that perfectly suited the salon culture of the French aristocracy. Their faces were idealized rather than psychologically penetrating – beautiful, charming and slightly artificial, like perfectly crafted masks for an elegant masquerade. Where Baroque had been monumental and serious, Rococo was elegant, witty, and frankly pleasure-seeking – exactly the kind of art that would appeal to wealthy merchants and nobles commissioning paintings for their private residences.

Following the French Revolution, the grandeur of the Baroque and Rococo traditions ceased to be fashionable. And the backlash to the Enlightenment's focus on rationality and reason came in the form of Romanticism, with its intense regard for the rugged awe of the natural world. 'Nature is a dictionary; one draws words from it,' announced Eugène Delacroix, whose *Self-Portrait* of circa 1837 (fig. 10) reveals a shadowy darkness and complex facial expression: furrowed brow, distracted gaze and unkempt hair.

The same fascination with faces as mirrors of inner character appeared in literature, too. In Emily Brontë's *Wuthering Heights* (1847). Heathcliff's face and body become the physical manifestation of the Yorkshire moors, the setting for the drama. Heathcliff

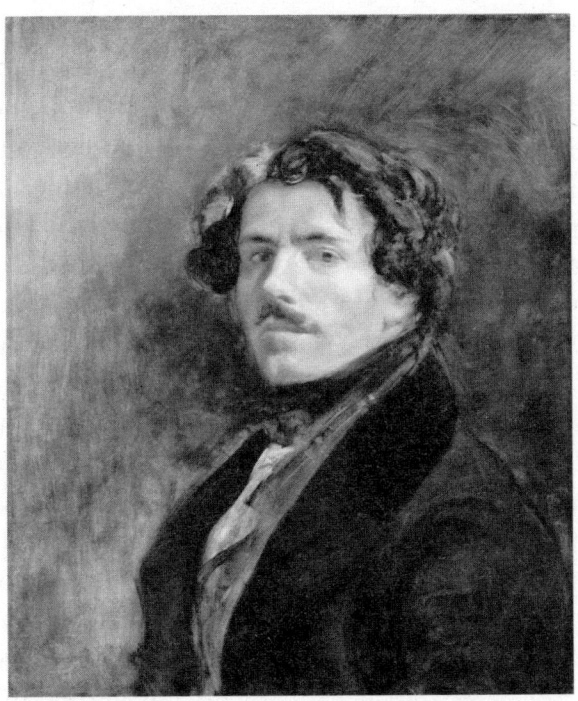

10. Eugène Delacroix, *Self-Portrait*, c, 1837.

is a 'dark-skinned gypsy', whose savagery is marked by 'two lines between [his] eyes; and those thick brows, that, instead of rising arched, sink in the middle, and that couple of black fiends, so deeply buried, who never open their windows boldly, but lurk glinting under them, like devil's spies.' The author was familiar with the work of the Swiss physiognomist and philosopher Johann Kaspar Lavater, who used physiognomy to show that a person's external features displayed their inner character, morality and destiny. As we will see in the following chapter, Lavater's work would soon make its way into criminal anthropology, evolutionary theory and eugenics.

By the end of the nineteenth century, artists and patrons worried less about realism in art, because photography could capture a person's likeness. Portrayals of the face were still expected to follow some essential truth, but it was increasingly unclear what that truth was. *The Scream* by the Norwegian artist Edvard Munch does away with any attempt at likeness and focuses on the impossibility of communicating a person's psychological state. Originally exhibited under the name *Der Schrei der Natur* (*The Scream of Nature*), the painting's agonized face is now one of the most iconic images in art.

There was a personal tale behind Munch's inspiration; he had been walking at sunset near to the asylum where his beloved sister Laura was incarcerated, and the blood-red of the sky seemed to echo the feelings in his own heart. But the work also reveals the anxieties of post-industrial Europe, with its radical social upheaval and industrial expansion. The horror on the face of the protagonist symbolizes the anonymity and facelessness of the modern world: Who are the men who are approaching the figure on the bridge? Why do they not hear the scream of nature? And why do our cries, and the corresponding cries of nature, go unheard?

Munch's work anticipated the Expressionist movement, and the concerns of Francis Bacon, who is famous for painting disturbing portraits. Although the trajectory of portraits since the fifteenth century had been towards likeness, and a specific human face, modernism changed that entirely. After the technological modernization of industrialization and mass production and the devastation of the First World War, everything that had seemed certain and stable in the West was turned on its head. And that included external reality. So, what was the role of the artist? For Bacon, that was simple:

> To me the mystery of painting today is how can appearance be made. I know it can be illustrated; I know it can be photographed. But how can this thing be made so that you catch the mystery of appearance within the mystery of making?

Many artists working after the First World War were concerned with the same question. There was a widespread disillusionment with traditional values in post-war Europe, while the combined forces of psychoanalysis and existentialism led to new, often fragmented and experimental forms. Movements like Dada and Surrealism were responses to the brutality and trauma of war, and Cubism fractured the picture plane into the texture of a broken mirror. By representing the same object from multiple viewpoints on a single canvas, Picasso highlighted the fractured nature of human experience.

In *The Weeping Woman*, for example, Picasso portrays the face of fellow artist Dora Maar across different planes, so that we see her from the side and from the front simultaneously. The rejection of realism and the chaotic rendering of the image suggest we might never be able to know the individual depicted or grasp their subjective identity. This is not a recognizable face, and yet it is recognizable on a different level; it seems to reflect the mind of the subject, which brings us closer to Bacon's 'mystery of appearance'.

Whatever we read in a human face, it seems to say, there is more going on beneath the surface. Despite the influence of physiognomy, the face is not a mirror of the mind at all.

We cannot really know what a person is feeling, or who they are, from the face as a structure. We might be able to determine clues from a person's behaviour, tone and demeanour that something isn't right, but can we determine what, precisely? To some extent a person is always locked inside their own consciousness.

It is no coincidence that these chaotic, disordered visions in art were produced soon after passports legally relied on the face as an index to a person's identity. Prior to the First World War, narrative descriptions of a person were as important as their visual image, and photographs were not mandatory. As we will see in the following chapter, photographic portraits became important during a time of war to track people's movements more efficiently. Yet at the same time as these likenesses were being produced, mechanized warfare was destroying soldiers' faces in trenches for the first time – and at an unimaginable rate and scale.

In this context, modern art forces us to consider the nature of our identity, and whether we are ever reducible to our face. What are we looking at when we look at a person? What defines our identity beyond what is on the surface? These questions hang in the air in Bacon's 'Pope' series, his paintings based on Velázquez's *Portrait of Pope Innocent X* (1650). Velázquez's Pope, Innocent X (Giovanni Battista Pamphilj), was head of the Catholic Church. But Bacon deliberately subverts the seventeenth-century reverence of Velázquez's work.

In *Study after Velázquez's Portrait of Pope Innocent X* (fig. 11), Bacon's figure wears the colours and symbols that we have long associated with the Catholic Church, with wealth and power. But Bacon tears away the layers of distance and appropriated authority; the stable ecclesiastical backdrop is replaced by a black void in which the figure of the Pope is seated not on a traditional throne, but in an apparent cage, with a series of vertical and horizontal lines suggesting imprisonment. The traditional purple and red robes are chaotically smeared and blurred.

The Pope's face is the most distorted part of the painting, his features stretched, his mouth open wide in a scream. This is a violent and tormented Pope, very different from the calm, serene personage of Velázquez's original painting. In other versions in the series, the Pope's face is reduced still further, until the figure is just a mouth, screaming into the void.

That what we see in a face can never reflect reality was a point

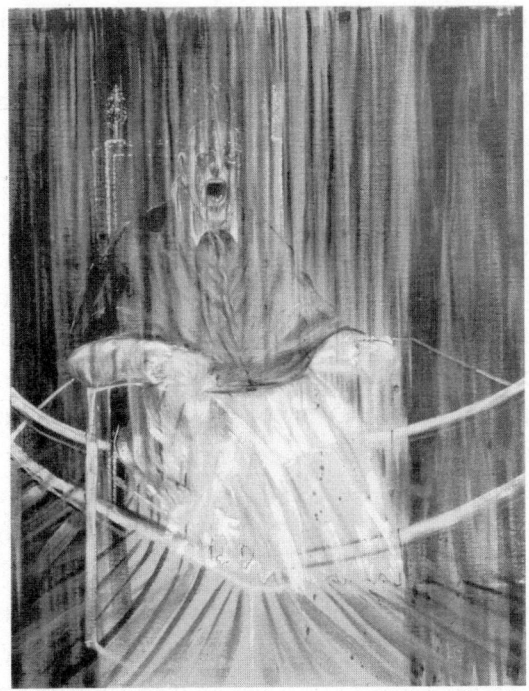

11. Francis Bacon, *Study after Velázquez's Portrait of Pope Innocent X*, 1953.

made, profoundly, and tragically, by the artist Bryan Charnley. He lived with paranoid schizophrenia; frustrated by his relative lack of success in the art world, and the impact of the medication he took for his mental illness, Charnley embarked on an experiment. He would stop taking his medication and create a series of self-portraits that showed what he saw in the mirror over time. His *Self-Portrait* series consists of seventeen paintings, each of which recorded an increasingly distorted version of his face, accompanied by a diary description of what it meant. Soon after he completed the last painting, Charnley killed himself.

Charnley's portraits bring together many important themes about portrayals of the face, from what a face is and does, to how portrayals change over time, and find an audience. But what a historical journey the face has been on! From a figurative representation on a cave wall, to a symbolic figurehead; from a faithful rendering of features to a fragmentation of the idea of the face and back to its figurative representation on a gallery wall, we have almost gone full circle.

If we broaden our inquiry, we could say that, too, about the circumstances of production and distribution. Formal portraiture was once undertaken by those and for those with skills and wealth; the skills were not recognized as 'art' in the modern sense until the Renaissance, but to be memorialized at all was a privilege. It was unthinkable for most people before the nineteenth century to have their faces portrayed.

Today, very few ordinary people have their faces immortalized in painting. But technological changes have channelled different ways for the face to be depicted and captured casually, routinely, formally and randomly, and not only for art, but also for humour, social connection, self-examination, legal identification, and much more.

The current ubiquity of the face was driven by the changes that underpinned the growth of formal portraiture. A focus on the nameable, recognizable, face in art paralleled and made visible the belief that the face alone is an indicator of selfhood; it is individualism writ large on the body.

As we will see in the following chapter, however, it was photography that democratized portrayals of the face, that made it conceivable today for anyone without training or wealth or art materials, or a large wall on which to hang their canvas, or large crowds to come and gaze upon it, to capture an image of their face, and to share that image with others.

Originating as a product of Victorian science, photography also picked up and ran with other beliefs that were seeded through the history of portraiture: that we can capture the essence of a person from their face, that some faces matter more than others, that beauty reflects the goodness of the soul, and that judging a person by their face is not only possible but desirable. Let's go back to October 1839 to find out more.

2.
Captured

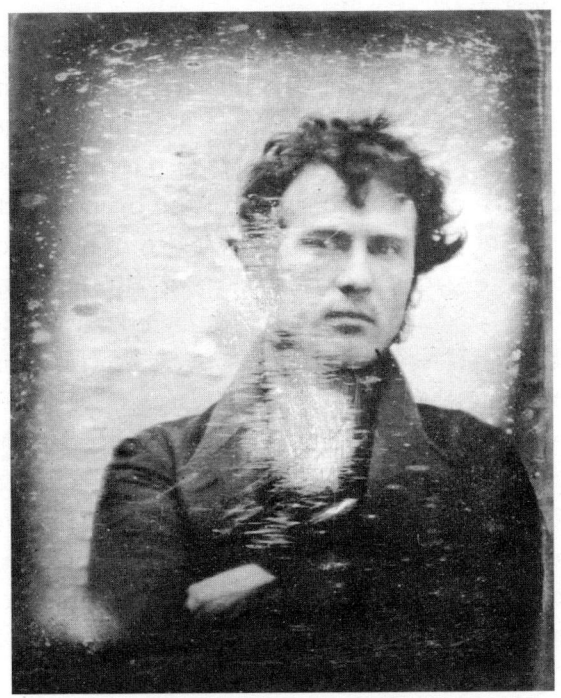

12. Robert Cornelius, *Self-Portrait*, 1839.

Picture yourself standing in a Philadelphia backyard on an October afternoon in 1839. The air carries the crisp promise of winter, and you're watching a man named Robert Cornelius fiddle with what looks like a tin box mounted on a makeshift stand. You are about to see history being made, with the creation of the first ever 'selfie'.

At thirty years old, Cornelius was running a successful lighting company, a family business, having previously specialized in his father's trade of silver plating and metal polishing. It was his friend and fellow inventor Joseph Saxton, a high-school teacher, who asked Cornelius to get involved in the process of photography, which at that time required a large degree of patience.

Then, early cameras produced daguerreotypes, which had hit the Philadelphia headlines earlier that same year because they enabled light from a camera obscura to be fixed through a chemical process. This was a transformative moment in technology, because it allowed images to be kept for ever. It wasn't, however, an easy or speedy affair.

To set up for a daguerreotype, you needed a silver-plated copper plate polished to a mirror finish. Next, you had to expose the plate to iodine until it turned yellow, before transferring it to a light-proof holder and exposing it to light in a large box camera. Then after the picture was taken, you had to fume the plate with mercury vapour to make the image visible, immerse it in salt to remove its sensitivity to light, and tone and enhance the image by using a solution of gold chloride to harden the plate.

Unlike modern photographs, each fragile daguerreotype was a precious, singular creation that demanded technical expertise and investment. Was it possible, Saxton asked Cornelius, to speed things up?

Cornelius figured that he could create a light-sensitive silver plate to shorten the set-up stage. And so it was that he ended up in his back yard, setting up that makeshift camera using a tin box and an opera-glass lens. Then, he stood in front of the camera.

The image Cornelius caught shows a dark-haired, clean-shaven, ruggedly handsome man, staring quizzically at the lens (fig. 12). He's wearing a dark frock coat, and standing just off-centre, as though caught off guard – though he would have had to stand patiently in the same place for at least nine minutes to get the exposure. On the back of the image, Cornelius scribbled a note: 'the first light Picture ever taken. 1839.'

By harnessing light to capture his own image, Cornelius's self-portrait marked the beginning of our modern obsession with documenting ourselves – and a revolution in how humans relate to their own faces.

Two months later, Cornelius took another photographic portrait, this time of his friend and collaborator, the physician Paul Beck Goddard (who, as an editor of medical books, saw clearly the teaching potential of photography). He collaborated with Goddard on using bromide to speed up the fixing process; rather than staying still for nine minutes, a sitter would only have to wait for two minutes – an eternity by today's impatient standards, but a vast improvement in the third decade of the nineteenth century.

Armed with this knowledge, Cornelius opened in Philadelphia one of the first portrait studios in America, where he captured the likenesses of other sitters, wealthy clients and family and friends. He subsequently opened another studio and became internationally known for his portraits. We don't know why Cornelius went back to his family business in 1843 – perhaps the business had too much competition from later studios, or perhaps he was content to focus on his latest invention: a solar lamp that ran cheaply on lard rather than the usual whale oil. The commercial success of his solar lamp made his family's lighting company the largest in the U.S.

But let's pause here to consider what photography represented to people experiencing it for the first time – those who flocked to the studios to have their images captured. The average cost of a daguerreotype was perhaps six dollars. At the same time a miniature painted in oil by a professional artist would cost around 250 dollars. For the first time ever, therefore, it was within the means of the masses to have their faces preserved for posterity.

This was a massive moment of democratization. For centuries, only the wealthy and powerful could afford to have their likenesses preserved. Suddenly, a shopkeeper, a teacher, a skilled craftsman could possess what had once been the exclusive privilege of kings and nobles: a permanent record of their face, proof of their existence that could outlast their mortal lives.

Today, Cornelius's single image is so important to the history of photography and American innovation that it is held in the special collections of the Library of Congress, along with his daguerreotype, lenses, papers, portraits of his children by other photographers, and a lock of his hair.

In popular culture, Cornelius's self-portrait is treated with less reverence. He could not have imagined that 200 years later it would be copied and colourized and sold online, or that his 'hotness' would be debated around the world by strangers. Most references to Cornelius, especially in digital media, refer to him simply as the creator of the first 'selfie'.

Technically, calling Cornelius's self-portrait a selfie is simply an anachronism: the term was first recorded in 2002 in the *Oxford English Dictionary* to mean a photograph you take of yourself, especially with a smartphone or webcam, and share via social media. The means of production and distribution built into today's digital world obviously did not exist in the 1830s.

But this *was* the first intentional photographic portrait. And it involved a very different type of skill and self-scrutiny to that we saw by Dürer and other portrait artists in the previous chapter. There was no established genre for Cornelius to be part of, nothing resembling the self-conscious performance of later photographic self-portraitists – such as David Hockney or Cindy Sherman.

There was also a vast chasm of difference between photography and the golden age of portraiture that took place between the fourteenth and seventeenth centuries, where commissioning and creating the image of a face depended on money, power and patronage. Back then, sitting for a portrait would have been an occasion; except for royals, people wealthy enough to afford to have a portrait painted would do it once, perhaps twice in their lifetime. And a portrait would not be circulated further than the guests who visited it *in situ*, or the suitors to whom it was sent.

By contrast, the average person today takes 450 selfies a year. Most of these are taken by younger generations, who are more used to curating facets of their lives to share. It's an extraordinary shift in thinking about how images of the face are produced and shared and valued. 'Reach' is everything to the modern selfie; the premise of influencer trends is that as many people should look at your image as possible, 'like' that image, and, by extension, value the self being portrayed.

This transformation reveals something profound about how we've come to understand faces and identity. When we capture a face with a camera, we are doing something different from what painters did when they produced a portrait. This is not just because photographic portraits are routine and most of us aren't declaring our status as rulers or leaders; it's also because we can change how we portray ourselves as often as our technology – and perhaps our companions' patience – allow. We might record moments of national importance, but we are far more likely to catch personal and even intimate moments, chasing perhaps the things that we know are fleeting – youth, beauty, love, time.

In selfies, the face can now be filtered, highlighted and posed beyond recognition and bear no relation to our own likeness. But if we don't like it, we can delete it from our mobile phones, our albums, our timelines. We curate our images without even being conscious of it. This casual relationship with image-making would have been incomprehensible to Cornelius and his contemporaries.

The speed, ease and availability of portraits today mean that the drive to capture an image can take priority over what is captured. Subtleties and nuance are lost if everything becomes a backdrop to the need to remember it. This is how we end up with inappropriately smiling faces in the most unlikely places: bomb sites; funerals; monuments and memorials, even the gas chambers of Auschwitz.

It seems fitting, then, that a much earlier entry for the meaning of 'selfy' was given in the *Oxford English Dictionary* in a 1643 letter written by Robert Baillie, the Church of Scotland minister and author: 'self-centred or selfish'.

But this is only one dimension of photography's impact on how we understand faces. There are two other, related aspects of capturing the face to think about in relation to this new technology. On the one hand, photography has played a key role in the history of portraiture – and contributed to, facilitated and informed the stories we tell about the world; It has enabled artists to create beautiful and emotive works that speak to essential truths about existence.

On the other hand, photography – once a means of self-reflection – could also be used for nefarious purposes. That aspect was reinforced by photography's association with transparency and truth. For Victorian scientists and bureaucrats seeking validation for ways to 'objectively' sort people into types and orders, photography was a vital tool; it has contributed more than any other technology to the classification of faces – as worthy or unworthy, beautiful or ugly, normal or pathological.

Both aspects of early photography were united by the theme of light. Victorian culture celebrated the bringing of light into darkness with lightness representing understanding, education, enlightenment, and progress, whereas darkness represented savagery, ignorance and immorality. To Victorian missionaries, busy converting 'natives' in far-flung lands, white faces shone like beacons; dark faces were frightening and dangerous. This story built on tropes that were in place long before Victorian science created racial hierarchies – many of them dating back to classical ideals of goodness and beauty that were found in Aristotle.

These deeply embedded metaphors of light and darkness profoundly influenced not just artistic depiction, but also the systemic categorization and treatment of diverse populations, against whom photography was a powerful tool.

Industrialists also wanted to end darkness, by lighting their factories cheaply and safely. Industrial capitalism couldn't be governed and limited by sunrise and sundown, and cheap tallow candles would have stunk out the linen factories and posed a fire hazard. By 1805, Philips and Lee's Cotton Mill in Manchester was able, by virtue of gas lamps, to remain open twenty-four hours a day – the first factory in England to do so. Entertaining at home was something that could be achieved with oil lamps too.

Light transformed the domestic interiors of the wealthy too; gas lighting in homes changed how individuals saw and looked at their faces, and the faces of others. I wonder, when candles cast a flattering glow, and mirrors weren't available, did we fret so much about how we looked? Combined with other material objects, like mirrors, which we will explore in the following chapter, artificial lighting fundamentally altered human self-perception – suddenly we could see ourselves and others with unprecedented clarity.

This was the social context of light and its uses when Cornelius created the 'first light picture ever taken'. His improvised kit came from a camera obscura (from the Latin, 'dark room'), whose principles were first described in fourth-century BCE China.

Originally a scientific instrument, the value to artists of the camera obscura became clear in the Renaissance. Consisting of a room, or a box, with an opening to allow light in, a camera obscura received light and projected an image of the outside world. Like the image formed in an eye's retina, the image was upside down; an angled mirror was used to reflect it the right way up.

With a camera obscura, scientists could look safely at solar eclipses, and artists, by sliding a thin piece of paper over a projected image and tracing it, could create facsimiles of the world around them. They were more interested in landscapes than faces, in part because the camera obscura was particularly good at sweeping images of perspective, as seen in the paintings of the Grand Canal in Venice made by Canaletto in the eighteenth century.

All this changed with the daguerreotype process, so named after its French inventor, Louis Daguerre, who guaranteed a 'truthful likeness' in portrait photography. Just a few months before Cornelius got involved, daguerreotypists in France had been inviting politicians and writers to their studios to publicize the photographic portrait to the masses. And though Cornelius opened his studio earlier, there were at least seventy photographic studios operating in New York City alone by 1850.

There was a huge public appetite for portrait photography, even though having your photograph taken was a horrible process. Before exposure time was shortened significantly by the work of Cornelius and others, your face would have to be powdered white, and your head held in a clamp. Your expression would need to be as fixed as your head, you couldn't blink, and you would probably become bored and uncomfortable quite quickly.

At the end of the century, the American politican and author Lucius E. Chittenden recalled being photographed in 1842:

> The operators rolled out what looked like an overgrown barber's chair with a ballot box attachment on a staff in front of it. I was seated in the chair and its Briarean arms seized me by the wrists, ankles, waist and shoulders. There was an iron bar which served as an elongation of the spine, with a cross bar in which the head rested, which held my head and neck as in a vice. Then, when I felt like a martyr in the embrace of the Nuremberg 'Maiden', I was told to assume my best Sunday expression, to fix my eyes on the first letter of the sign of a beer saloon opposite, and not to move or wink on pain of 'spoiling the exposure'. One of the executioners said I must not close my eyes or move for ten minutes, at the end of which he would signal by a tap on the ballot box. The length of that cycle was too awful for description.

This vivid account shows how photography transformed the human face into an object to be disciplined, controlled and artificially maintained.

In *The Evolution of Photography*, the Victorian photographer John Werge tells the story of a woman who travelled miles to see an itinerant daguerreotypist. Once she was sitting in front of the camera and the lens uncapped, the daguerreotypist excused himself, to have a smoke perhaps, or to check his schedule. When he got back, he found the woman relieved that the sitting was over. She headed back to her home in Yorkshire, and the daguerreotypist started the developing process. To his bafflement:

> The ground, the wall and the chair whereon she sat, were all visible, but the image of the lady was not; and the operator was completely puzzled, if not alarmed . . . The mystery was, however, explained in a few days, when the lady called for her portrait, for she admitted

that she got up and walked about as soon as he left her, and only sat down again when she heard him returning. The necessity of remaining before the camera was not recognised by that sitter.

Despite these problems, and the cost and fragility of images, daguerreotypes were popular until the next innovation came along: *cartes de visite*, or visiting cards, which were much cheaper, not just because they were smaller, but also because they allowed eight images to be taken on a glass plate, before the negative was cut into individual portraits to be mounted on cards. With the *cartes de visite*, patented by André Adolphe-Eugène Disdéri in 1854, posing for photographs became easier and more comfortable, and the circulation of images for professional and personal use increased.

Cartes de visite were an advance on script-only calling cards, a sort of cross between baseball cards (also produced from the 1860s) and the profile photos we find on Facebook: they were swapped between friends and visitors, and family albums became a fixture of Victorian drawing rooms.

The cards expanded the mass market for photographs and marked a crucial moment in the history of the face: suddenly, people could have multiple photographic versions of themselves to use for different audiences. The idea that you might curate various versions of yourself through imagery, now so familiar to us through social media, has its roots in these small Victorian cards.

Celebrity culture as we know it today didn't exist, but we can see tentative steps in that direction by studios who used images of well-known people such as Charles Dickens to promote their services. Dickens himself had a particular interest in the face; the physical appearance of his characters was based on classical physiognomic ideas, which the Victorians reinvigorated with prejudices old and new. In Oliver Twist, 'the Jew' Fagin, is a 'loathsome reptile' with a large nose and red hair, and the thieving Artful Dodger was physically dirty, with 'bowlegs and little, sharp, ugly eyes'. In life, however, Dickens recognized that the camera was kinder to some people than to others: 'We do not all come out of the photographic studio alike unhappy. There are those to whom the process does justice, as well as those to whom it does injustice.'

Many people worried they did not look good in photographs – much as they do today. So much so that by 1928 the Victorian word 'photogenic' (which in the 1830s meant 'produced by light') started meaning 'photographing well'.

Of course, people have always wanted to look their best in photographic portraits, especially when they were taken as an act of remembrance. During the American Civil War soldiers would leave a personalized *carte de visite* as a token for their wife or lover, and these images sometimes served broader purposes, even becoming powerful tools for propaganda. Post-mortem portraits were also common. Taking a photograph of a loved one propped up in a coffin, or posed alongside living siblings, seems very odd by today's standards, but it was a popular Victorian ritual of death. Before photography, people had created paintings and drawings of the dead, taken locks of hair to wear in lockets and rings, and made death masks in wax.

Many of these practices came from earlier times but the Victorians excelled in *memento mori* (from Latin, meaning 'remember you must die'). Queen Victoria herself released photos of the corpse of her husband, Prince Albert, lying on his deathbed in the Blue Room at Windsor Castle. The prince's body is covered by bedsheets, his pale face is in repose, and a bandage wrapped around his head holds his jaw closed.

Photography offered a way to hold on to the faces of the dead in a manner more precise and lasting than any previous technology. In an era of high mortality rates, especially for children, these images served as precious talismans of love and loss.

By the First World War such images were falling from favour – perhaps because photography was accessible enough that people could be photographed in life; or because societal attitudes towards death had shifted and became more medicalized, meaning that dead bodies were increasingly managed by medical institutions and moved to mortuaries. But it might also have been that the First

World War caused so much death, nobody needed to be further reminded of it.

So, what drove people to photograph the living? Just because technology becomes available, that doesn't guarantee its popularity. Who remembers the ill-fated invention, the Sinclair C5?

One of the reasons for the success of photography was peer pressure; if other people were doing it, why not join in? And it continued painted portraiture's increasing popularity in earlier centuries, democratizing an art form that had previously been the privilege of the wealthy by making it available to the middling sorts.

With an increasing number of portraits came increasing diversity of purpose. On the domestic front, portraits were made for families, for lovers, for grieving mothers, for friends; on the commercial front, by the end of the nineteenth century, images of women were being used to promote consumer goods.

Companies like Kodak realised that sex sells. Their models predated the barrage of famous faces that started appearing in the early twentieth century, as Hollywood movie stars loomed large on big screens, emoting madly, and celebrity magazines appeared, full of backstage gossip and innuendo.

A thriving underground market also developed for erotic and nude *cartes de visite*. These 'boudoir' cards were produced secretly and varied widely – some were just mildly suggestive whereas others showed full nudity or even sexual acts. The huge demand for these images likely helped fuel the rapid growth of photography, continuing a familiar pattern where adult content has driven the adoption of new technologies throughout history – from the printing press to the internet.

'Cartomania', as the interest in *cartes de visite* had become known, faded out of fashion when newer technologies such as the box camera emerged. From 1888, you could take a photograph at home without training, skills or any other equipment if you bought George Eastman's Kodak camera. The word Kodak was apparently a deliberate onomatopoeic rendering of the click made by a camera shutter – a sound that will mean nothing to a generation brought up on iPhones.

This shift from professional studios to personal cameras resents another crucial development in our relationship with our faces; they became something we could document casually, spontaneously, without ceremony or special occasion.

Earlier, photography had also evolved as a tool for classification and categorization, and these were themes that mattered hugely to Victorians. Unlike portraiture, photography seemed to offer an 'objective' rendering of a face. This truth value gave it another important role in Victorian culture. Anthropologists, criminologists and scientists of all kinds were united in the quest to objectively measure, count and classify human beings at home and in the colonies.

Rapid industrial, urban and international expansion required bureaucratic systems of administration and regulation – everything, and everyone, needed to be standardized to manage the growing complexity of society and economy. This was especially the case in urban and colonial environments, where those in power feared anonymity, crime and lawlessness.

The need for order was accompanied by scientific interest in cataloguing humans, building on the eighteenth-century taxonomies developed by the Swedish naturalist Carl Linnaeus. His system included racial categories such as *Europaeus albus* (European white), *Americanus rubescens* (American reddish), *Asiaticus fuscus* (Asian tawny) and *Africanus niger* (African black).

In his *Systema Naturae* (1735), Linnaeus attached behavioural and cultural characteristics to each group of people:

1. *Homo sapiens Americanus* (Native American): reddish, choleric, obstinate, content, free. Paints himself with fine red lines. Ruled by custom.
2. *Homo sapiens Europaeus* (European): white, sanguine, muscular. Gentle, inventive, wears tight clothing. Governed by laws.

3. *Homo sapiens Asiaticus* (Asian): tawny, melancholic, stiff. Severe, haughty, avaricious. Covered with loose garments. Governed by opinions.
4. *Homo sapiens Africanus* (African): black, phlegmatic, relaxed. Cunning, indolent, negligent. Anoints himself with grease. Governed by caprice.

However absurd and offensive these categories are today, they had a long and lasting impact. They have been used to define different 'races', the biological layering that Victorian scientists added to geographic and visible differences.

Photography allowed permanent images of people's faces and bodies to be captured. Those images were lined up and compared so that every aspect of a person could be catalogued and placed in a hierarchy: height and colouring; cranium and brain size; nose length and width; lip width; brow shape; eye size and shape, and more besides.

Bear in mind that the Victorians inherited from classical philosophers like Aristotle the flawed idea that a person's outside reflects their inside. Victorian bureaucrats and scientists borrowed from those ideas to make 'scientific' distinctions and links between people's appearance, personality and morality. Those distinctions confirmed two basic imperialist presumptions: that white men were at the top of the human tree, and that truth was evident in every aspect of a person's appearance, if you knew where to look.

What a boon this was for the growing institutions of Victorian culture, at home and in their overseas territories – for schools, prisons, asylums and hospitals! These places needed to identify and classify individuals quickly and shared a bureaucratic desire to sort people into groups.

Why does this matter? Well, the unfounded idea that character, intelligence and moral worth could be read from the face moved from philosophical theory to become the basis of decisions about education, employment, imprisonment and immigration for millions of people. And, as we will see, the idea remains with us today.

The Face

In the past, facial distinctiveness – that is, the fact of looking like a named individual – did not matter for most people, as we saw in our discussion of portraiture; and there was no bureaucracy in place to track the individual identity of every peasant. But what happens when those peasants begin to move around into towns, to break laws and threaten social order? How did the authorities know if the person they arrested had committed a crime, and how could they overcome the poorer sort of recidivist criminals who they were convinced lurked around every corner? How could they know, given increased mobility, that a person was who they said they were? How could they anticipate, from a glance, a person who was likely to break the law? And what could be done to protect civilized society from degenerating into a nation of deviants?

Such questions were at the forefront of the minds of the 'better sort' in Victorian culture. There was a lot at stake in the urbanizing, commercial world of the nineteenth century.

Consider the famous story of the medieval French peasant Martin Guerre, impersonated by a stranger who lived with Martin's wife for several years before being found out. Nobody could *prove*, since there were no recorded images of the peasant's face, that Guerre was an imposter – until the 'real' Guerre turned up.

The spectre of Martin Guerre was in the minds of many Victorians when Roger Tichborne, heir to the Tichborne baronetcy, was lost, in 1854, in a shipwreck. His mother refused to believe her twenty-five-year-old son and heir was dead. When rumours circulated that Tichborne had found his way to Australia, she put advertisements in newspapers there, offering a large reward. Twelve years later, a butcher from Wagga Wagga came forward to say that he was Roger Tichborne. The claimant had none of the manners and bearing one might associate with an aristocrat of Victorian England, and he was much fatter than Roger had been. Nevertheless, the man was embraced by Roger's mother as her son, perhaps because she was desperate to believe he was alive.

Other family members were not convinced, and as determined to expose the fraud as Martin Guerre's relatives had been. In both cases, money was at stake. The resulting court cases were drawn out and bitter and, despite the claimant campaigning for popular support, a court declared that he was not Roger Tichborne, but Arthur Orton, a butcher's son and originally from Wapping.

Orton was sentenced to fourteen years in prison as punishment for his fraud. However, as with other so-called 'pretenders' (including two claimants to the throne of England in the fifteenth century, Lambert Simnel and Perkin Warbeck, the latter pretending to be the younger of the two Princes in the Tower), Orton's punishment did not end speculation; a popular movement arose to champion his cause.

How did one truly know who someone was, in the absence of scientific evidence such as DNA, and with no recorded visual identifiers? Most of us would say that we know a lover, a child, a friend, by signs other than their face – we know people by their scent, their voice, their touch, the way that they move, or tilt their head when asked a question, by what they remember and know and share.

But none of these subjective experiences could be counted by bureaucrats, or known by strangers, and none of these things were comparable between people as objectively as wrapping a tape measure around a person's head or analysing their mugshot. Just one daguerreotype existed of the real Roger Tichborne, and it was a single, unclear image, which didn't help at all in determining whether the claimant from Wagga Wagga was the lost boy or a criminal chancer. Personal identity, even in a rigidly class-based society, was vulnerable to attack.

The resultant anxiety about identity and impersonation reveals something crucial about the Victorian moment: as society became more mobile and anonymous, the face became the primary anchor of individual identity. The terror wasn't just that someone might steal your property or position – it was that your very self could be stolen, that someone else could inhabit your identity so completely that even your own family might be deceived.

No wonder that the spectre of the 'doppelgänger' became popular in the Victorian period; fiction played with the idea that a person might have a double – that one's place in the world could be snatched away at any moment. Sometimes this idea tapped into much older fears of the supernatural and of twins – the closeness of Roderick and Madeline in Edgar Allan Poe's *The Fall of the House of Usher*, for instance, echoes the shared destiny of Castor and Pollux in Roman mythology (Kastor and Polydeuces for the Greeks).

In the Victorian period, however, the doppelgänger was more profoundly linked to social expectation and a person's struggle with their subconscious. We find that in Fyodor Dostoevsky's *The Double*, and in Poe's short story 'William Wilson', which was published in 1839 – the same year that Cornelius stepped in front of the camera lens.

The story is about a young man, William, from a 'misty looking village' in England, who goes away to school, where he meets another boy with the same name and the same appearance, born on the same date. Over time, the boy dresses and moves more like William until even the 'lineaments' of his face become identical. William is haunted by his double for years, and that double even prevents him from gratifying his desires. Eventually, William stabs and kills the double, only then realizing that he has killed himself.

The doppelgänger wasn't invented by Victorians; the word – which means 'double goer' in German – was coined in the eighteenth century, and it builds on that much longer mythological history of paranormal spirits and evil twins.

By the nineteenth century, doppelgängers were mostly discussed in symbolic rather than literal terms; the reason why they became more associated with a person's social and psychological status was that Victorian culture valued a respectable public image. This could lead to a psychological disconnect between a person's true self and their outward persona – further fuelling the idea of a hidden 'double'. As a literary device, doppelgängers helped writers explore the inner darkness of characters – which was an endless source of fascination for Victorians.

Sometimes the disparity between a person's outward appearance and interior reality was dangerous – as in Robert Louis Stevenson's

Strange Case of Dr Jekyll and Mr Hyde or Oscar Wilde's *The Picture of Dorian Gray* – both of which showed that what we see is not always what we get.

We still worry about doppelgängers, despite DNA evidence and visual proofs, from photography to CCTV. And fiction is still concerned with how individual any of us really are – from Patricia Highsmith's novel, and later film, *The Talented Mr Ripley*, and John Lutz's thriller *SWF Seeks Same* (made into the hit movie *Single White Female*), to more recent Netflix series: *Echoes* and *Triptych*. But in modern versions of the doppelgänger story, we worry mostly about the reliability of the systems that promise to authenticate us; passports can be forged, babies swapped, DNA cloned, faces and voices deepfaked.

Such worries were not on the minds of most Victorians, who had faith in the objective and the bureaucratic – at least more faith than they had in the emotional and the subjective, both characteristics shared by children, women and 'inferior races'. Victorian bureaucrats believed that technological systems would improve the ad hoc, sporadic attempts at social regulation found in earlier periods; this is why the rulers of European cities, in classifying human faces, used the same methods and criteria as anthropologists working in the colonies.

Why faces? Why not hands, or gait, or habit? The simplest explanation is that the face was more routinely observable, harder to change and easier to describe. It couldn't be discarded or hidden if you were on the run.

Before the sixteenth century, your clothes, accent, behaviour and manners might mark you out. It is hard to imagine now, but for centuries, sumptuary legislation (from the Latin, meaning laws that regulated consumption) governed what clothes and even colours a person could wear, as well as what people ate and bought. In fifteenth-century England, 'royal purple' (purple, crimson, reds and royal blue) could only be worn by royalty or the clergy. Sable, ermine and velvet could only be worn by knights and lords, while yeomen and squires could wear damask and satin, but only if they made more than £40 a year. In Elizabeth I's reign – to stimulate wool markets, as well as to make workmen visible – all men and boys over six years old, except for the wealthy and people of degree, had to wear flat woollen caps on Sundays and public holidays.

It was possible to separate people out like this in a hierarchical system where everyone knew their place, and most people had only one set of clothes. It was not possible in the developing consumer economy of the eighteenth century, when more goods were available, and ordinary people cared more what they looked like.

Other than people flouting the sumptuary laws, which was increasingly common, the behaviour and manners of the wealthy could be copied – using the conduct manuals that sprang up in English, French and German, telling people how 'the mannered' might act and speak and behave. This levelling of appearance was troubling to people in power, who wanted to be able to tell people apart; what if identity could be slipped on and off like a frock coat?

When everything else was up for grabs and changeable, the face became the last reliable indicator of who someone 'really' was. This marked a fundamental change in how society understood and recorded individual identity.

Before photography took off in the 1840s, prison governors wrote down the physical characteristics of men and women they took into custody. They recorded a criminal's name, place of origin, date of birth, the name of the judge who sent them down, and observable information such as complexion, stature, hair colour and identifying marks. Under 'marks', they might note the colour of a convict's eyes, or whether they were bald or freckled, or had a scar. Or they might record that a person had small or large eyes, a big head, a long or broad nose.

This presented a problem for the Victorian bureaucrats; how could such descriptions be used to identify a person? How broad is a broad nose? At what point does a head become big?

The rising science of biometrics, which was part and parcel of Victorians' desire for measurement, offered a solution. Sorting criminals into groups based on their appearance was no different from identifying specimens for a museum according to genus, or measuring civilization in different races as defined by Linnaeus.

It could go even further: Francis Galton, who coined 'eugenics' in 1883 (from the Greek *eu* for good and *genesis* for birth), suggested that if you could identify who the degenerates were by appearance, you could stop them from breeding.

Galton was influenced by his cousin Charles Darwin, whose book *On the Origin of Species* was published in 1859. Many Victorians were outraged by Darwin's claims of a common primate ancestor, and he was often lampooned by cartoonists, who put his recognizable face, with its long beard, balding head, bushy eyebrows and serious expression, on the body of a chimp.

Galton was interested not only in Darwin's theory of evolution, but also in the potential of that theory for improving civilization. The Chinese, he suggested, should move to Africa to weed out Africans, and closer to home, degenerates and inferiors should be sterilized so that they couldn't have children.

Galton's views influenced ideology about 'uncivilized tribes' and peoples. 'I hate people with slit eyes and pigtails,' said the British Prime Minister Sir Winston Churchill, who was caricatured as a bulldog in the British press. 'I don't like the look of them or the smell of them.' Sadly, comments by Prince Philip (on the 'slitted eyes' of the Chinese in the 1980s) and Boris Johnson (on the 'watermelon smiles' of Black people in 2002) show the lingering influence of such derogatory language – even on people who should know better.

In pursuit of perfection, the Nazis carried out at least 400,000 forced sterilizations before 1939, and the practice spread to Japan, Denmark and Sweden. In the U.S., 70,000 sterilizations were forced on people who were 'mentally deficient', deaf, blind, or diseased. Eugenicists also aimed at 'promiscuous women', minorities and the poor. Eugenics still has influence in the twenty-first century – from the white nationalist 'Great Replacement' conspiracy theory to complex ethical debates about whether and how genetic editing might prevent disability.

This grim trajectory reveals how photography and facial analysis became tools not just of identification, but of systematic oppression. The apparent objectivity of the camera made it seem scientific, neutral, truthful – when it was being used to reinforce existing prejudices and create new forms of discrimination.

Explicit in the work of Francis Galton, and implicit in right-wing propaganda, is the idea that you can judge a book by its cover; that facial features, as Aristotle had said, showed who a person was.

The question was – what kind of organization or process was best to capture and use that data? Before he set up the Galton Laboratory, Galton travelled to Paris to meet a police officer who believed he had the answer.

Alphonse Bertillon, son of a French statistician, had taken to measuring the body, head and face through the science of anthropometry (meaning simply: human measurements). 'Bertillonage', as his system became known, was used across France and in several other countries. It involved each part of the criminal's body – their height, head length, arm span, sitting height, left middle finger and little finger length, forearm length, ear length – being measured and recorded on an identification certificate.

Bertillon's plan, as set out in his *Identification Anthropométrique*, was to 'fix the human personality, give to each human being an identity, a certain individuality, durable, invariable, always recognizable and easily demonstrable'. After all, the body could not lie – could it?

Yes it could, since people did not always interpret the body in the same way. Bertillon's fame and reputation were such that he became head of France's Service d'identité judiciaire. But the system kept running into difficulties – two people measuring a person's forearm in relation to their ear length and the little finger of their left hand might not come up with the same numbers. And each police unit, even across France, ended up using the system differently. Some of the categories used were also subjective – lips could be pouting, thick or thin; beards could be supple, curly, frizzy or very frizzly – so facial descriptions needed to be supplemented.

Could photography be the answer? Bertillon didn't think so. He toyed with accompanying his written descriptions with mugshots, which are still used today. But he was frustrated by the results. His system of visual measurements proved inaccurate when used alongside photographs of criminals. And there was a problem with the sheer scale of numbers – the Parisian police alone amassed 100,000 photographs of criminals; how would anyone go through those photographs to match them up with the detailed descriptions of hundreds of people arrested daily? Besides, Bertillon said, a person could look completely different in two different photographs!

For Bertillon the measurements of the body were more persuasive, as he tried to convince Galton when he visited Paris. By way of illustration, Bertillon took Galton's measurements and his photograph, which showed him turned out in cravat and waistcoat (fig. 13).

Galton, in turn, was unconvinced. He went on to develop a different system, based on a facial shorthand. This 'Classification of Portraits' was published in *Nature*, where he wrote of his experiments to 'define the facial particularities of persons' through the careful measurement of 'persons, families and races'. It should be

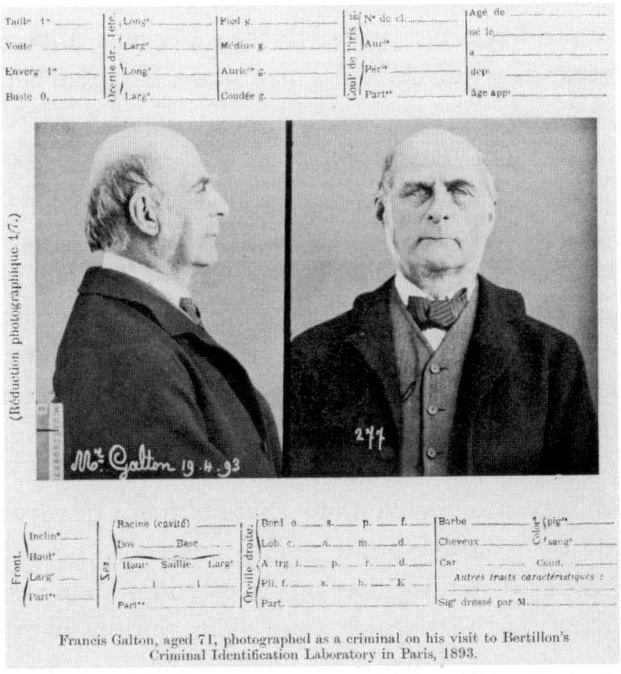

13. Alphonse Bertillon, Mugshot of Francis Galton, 1893.

possible, Galton argued, to 'lexiconise' portraits, especially profiles, in the same way that dictionaries sort words in alphabetical order.

Galton's language of the face was based on the idea that every face, especially in profile, could be differentiated by the relationship between six features: the chin; the lower and upper lip; the hollow between the upper lip and the nose; the nose; the hollow between the nose and the brow. It was possible to produce a series of quantifiable, comparable numbers from these six points, Galton claimed, though his scheme failed to take off.

Galton's composite photography proved more popular; he pioneered a technique of superimposing a series of portraits on top of one another, looking for some shared characteristic that would help him understand faces as a type, as well as an individual. Was there a 'criminal look' that might help detect deviants, even before they committed a crime?

This question had been asked before, by the eighteenth-century physiognomist Lavater – who you might remember influenced Emily Brontë when she created the characters in *Wuthering Heights*. He claimed falsely, as Aristotle had done, that deviance could be read in the face.

Lavater had his Victorian equivalent in one of Galton's friends, Cesare Lombroso, an Italian criminologist and author of *L'uomo delinquente* (*Criminal Man*; 1876). Like Galton, Lombroso was inspired by Charles Darwin's evolutionary theories; offensive as it is to modern readers, he understood evolution to explain how criminals – like people of colour – were 'throwbacks' to some earlier phase of human evolution. We will look more closely into this connection in chapter seven.

What Bertillon did for criminology in France, Lombroso did in Italy with his invention of the 'criminal man'. Using autopsy evidence and comparative photography, Lombroso plotted supposed similarities between the physiology of criminal offenders and 'primitive humans', both of which were likened to monkeys and apes. Conveniently, the atavistic 'born criminal' could be detected by the measurements of the face.

There were identifiable criminal facial characteristics according to Lombroso. This included 'sugarloaf' shaped skulls (so named after refined white sugar produced by slave labour and prepared in cone-shaped moulds). Lombroso's criminals also had heavy jaws (rather like Victorian models of Neanderthals), receding brows and scant beards. Their heads tended to be small, their mouths fleshy, they had bumps on the back of the skull and around the ear, wrinkles on the forehead, large sinuses, a receding hairline, big eye sockets with deep-set eyes, high cheekbones, large incisors, bushy eyebrows, a beaked or flat nose, a weak chin, a thin neck and an insensitivity to pain.

Imagine how this pseudo-scientific cataloguing must have felt to those subjected to it. Picture yourself being examined, measured, photographed and categorized according to these arbitrary standards – your very humanity reduced to a checklist of supposedly criminal features. This wasn't mere theory; such ideas influenced real judicial decisions, prison sentences and immigration policies.

Classifying people into groups wasn't new – it was the basis of Galenic theory, which separated people into humoral types: choleric, phlegmatic, sanguine and melancholic. But the humours were holistic, and included the mind, body and soul into a broader concept of balance. Because of the heat-based nature of physiology (men being hotter), men were angrier and women sadder. There were physical differences because of humours: women's hair was longer whereas men's was burned up by their heat. And similarly, people in hotter climates like Spain were presumed to have hotter tempers, whereas those living in colder climates like the U.K. tended towards the melancholic. Such were the ways that culture was overlaid onto the physical structure of the body.

But the formula of the Victorians was supposedly 'scientific', as well as being rigidly hierarchical and fixed. You could change your humour in the Galenic model, by bloodletting, purging, changing your diet, all of which affected the balance of the humours. Feeling sad? Stop eating dark meat, such as hare, which produced melancholic humours. A little manic? Indulge in a little bloodletting. Angry and resentful? Eat cold food.

By contrast, in Victorian science your identity and your habits were fixed. In anthropological texts, physiological treatises, museum dioramas, medical casebooks and human zoos, comparative physiognomy justified white supremacy and colonial rule. And photography did not simply reflect those hierarchies, it helped create them.

Some African Americans explicitly rejected this racial positioning by setting up their own studios – as the Goodridge Brothers did in Pennsylvania in 1847. Although born enslaved and indentured, the parents of the Goodridge Brothers, William C. and Evalina Goodridge, became successful entrepreneurs in Pennsylvania. Their children, William and Wallace, set up a studio that thrived until the 1920s. Their portraits celebrated individualism and community among African Americans. The symbolic importance of their work deserves more attention from historians than it has received, especially to counteract the many portrayals of Black faces to represent savages, minstrels and slaves.

It might surprise you that Frederick Douglass, the social reformer, abolitionist, writer and statesman who fled slavery, sat for some 160 images during his lifetime – more than any other nineteenth-century man, including President Lincoln. Douglass knew how valuable photography was in telling a story and offering an alternative to the propaganda of white power and Black subordination. In an image from 1847 he appears handsome, well-groomed and serious, a deliberate challenge to the racist stereotypes of grinning, happy slaves, or dirty, uneducated labourers.

These acts of resistance matter because photography was given a truth value that other technologies did not have. The Victorians prioritized sight over all other senses; for them, seeing was believing. Photography and science worked hand in hand to construct a version of 'objective' face values that are still influential in defining what is beautiful, as well as what is deviant, undesirable and uncivilized.

Photography did this seamlessly because it followed the conventions of traditional portraiture; and because for those who were not branded criminal or deviant, it was an innocuous, fun and yet important means of recording their everyday lives. This process echoes how some people happily give up their facial biometric data today, in exchange for a face filter that turns back the years. If it's fun, how can it be harmful?

Photography did not merely capture and catalogue faces; it also enabled them to be tracked. To understand photography's role in identification systems, it is worth comparing it to its contemporary alternative: fingerprinting. Historians of surveillance technology focus most often on fingerprinting, a method that emerged from colonial contexts. In the 1860s, British colonial administrators found fingerprinting more reliable than photography for distinguishing between Indian subjects, as they struggled to differentiate individual faces – a phenomenon now understood as the Other Race Effect, which we will examine in chapter five.

However, fingerprinting had significant limitations that made photography a more powerful tool for mass surveillance. Fingerprinting could not be performed instantly or at a distance in the way that one might look at and recognize a face. It required direct physical contact, specialized equipment and trained operators. Most importantly, fingerprinting was more invasive than photography, requiring the subject's cooperation or coercion. This invasiveness may explain why such techniques were more readily implemented in colonial territories like India, where subjects had fewer protections, than in European contexts where citizens possessed greater rights. Photography, by contrast, offered identification at scale – images could be taken quickly, reproduced cheaply and circulated widely, creating new possibilities for tracking individuals across time and space.

And so, it was the face that was used by modern state systems as they started to identify and track taxpayers, patients, suspects, travellers and soldiers.

Passport photographs became mandatory during and after the First World War. Before that, there was no international standard for passports at all, though many countries had developed some kind of travel documentation as travel became more widespread. Unlike modern-day passports or visas, which are issued by a nation state, early modern travel documents (often referred to as 'safe conducts') were issued by the authorities of a specific region. Travellers showed them to the guards posted at borders to prove that the bearer had permission to travel.

Formal passports had become more common after the French Revolution, a time of great social and political unrest – there is nothing like military conflict to strengthen authorities' interest in known and unknown faces. This relaxed in the mid-nineteenth century, but the First World War made it more important for states to know who was leaving or entering their countries. In 1914, the United States made photographs compulsory for passports, with Britain following in 1915. This wasn't the first use of photographs in travel documents, but by 1920 they were internationally standardized. Early passport photographs followed *carte de visite* conventions, showing people lounging or posed with friends, but by 1926 they had to be 'full face', hatless, and focused solely on identifying features.

Think about what this standardization meant. No longer could you present yourself as you chose to be seen – lounging elegantly, surrounded by family, or in your finest clothes. The state demanded a specific type of image: direct, unadorned, focused solely on facial features that could be used for identification and control. This shift marked the beginning of our modern relationship between faces and bureaucratic power.

Today an identity card or travel document without a photograph of the face is unthinkable. And we expect a face to reflect a person's unique individuality, though we are also interested in family resemblances, and how we might share a nose shape, an eye colour, an expression with our parents or grandparents.

The current fashion for genealogy perpetuates the importance of facial heredity, as do the ways we romanticize the past through digital culture, in 'face apps' that invite viewers to see themselves as nineteenth-century literary heroines or figures in Renaissance paintings. And while many of us have concerns about privacy and identity theft, for most people these technologies have appropriated the trust we used to have in photography, when there was a single person behind the camera, rather than a multimillion-pound industry trading our biometric data.

This is true, too, of the facial-recognition technologies (FRT) routinely used in shopping centres to determine, based on a shopper's 'look' and facial expression, whether they are there to shop or steal. And rather as Victorian scientists pondered over criminal faces, modern facial-recognition systems perpetuate racial stereotypes. We know that the algorithms of FRT are biased so that people of colour, and women, are routinely misidentified. Even so, these systems continue to be widely used without appropriate regulations.

Perhaps we are so casual about our data because we now take for granted that the face represents our legal and social selves. And perhaps we are so reluctant to address algorithmic bias because many of our technologies originated in Victorian prejudices and presumptions.

Even colour film (pioneered by the chemist James Clerk Maxwell in the 1860s and used in popular photography from the 1960s) has been calibrated on white skin.

This means that if customers once sent their Kodak film off to be developed in a lab, those photos would have been checked for colour, shadows and light against the skin of a 'Shirley card'. This was the image of a white brunette (who, possibly apocryphally, was once a Kodak employee). If Shirley looked good in the developing process, it meant the shadows, light and colour were correct. In the 1990s images of Latina or Black women began to be used on some versions of the 'Shirley card', but since digital photography appeared at the same time, all cards fell out of favour.

What changed things? There were complaints from chocolate and furniture manufacturers in the 1960s and 1970s that Kodak weren't getting the right brown tones on their products, according to some researchers. Fujifilm improved the colours used in Black skin tone in the 1980s, they obliquely promoted the film as being 'able to photograph the details of a dark horse in lowlight'.

We are a long way from equity, and in many parts of the world white faces are still seen, and prioritized, as the norm. Digital technology still struggles with dark skin tones, and in 2015 Google's face-recognition system infamously captioned images of Black people as 'Gorillas'.

All technology is developed and implemented within flawed human systems, and this includes our biometric focus on the face. In the early twenty-first century, the International Civil Aviation Organization (ICAO) approved a new standard for passports using facial recognition and biometrics. There was no widespread or public consultation on this; the technology was rolled out quickly in the aftermath of the 9/11 terrorist attacks on the World Trade Center in New York and elsewhere in the U.S. Even without that motivation, it is habitual today to equate an individual face with a specific citizen in ways that would have been unimaginable before portrait photography.

Today, most of us are also used to looking at faces, and having our faces looked at, even if there are complex power dynamics as to who is doing the looking, and who is being looked at. We crop people out of photographs digitally, as once we did physically, angrily, with a pair of scissors, perhaps after a bad break-up. We like the way we look in some photographs more than others; very few people are happy with the sullen image in their passports, stripped of any character or emotional expression. Many of us can't bear how we look in photographs. The image differs from how we feel. Mirrors reverse our faces, and we grow used to that reversed image. Photographs show us as others see us – unreversed – which can feel unsettling.

Mirrors and cameras have a lengthy history, with one another, and with light. Remember how the daguerreotypist had to polish a sheet of silver-plated copper to a mirror finish? Many early cameras used mirrors to project images and capture light (Digital Single-Lens Reflex – DSLR – cameras still do). And the owners of wealthy households in medieval Venice were as likely to use mirrors for reflecting light into dim chambers as to scrutinize their appearance in those mirrors. This interrelationship between the mirror and the camera was metaphorical as well as literal; in 1859 the American physician and writer Oliver Wendell Holmes Sr called the camera 'the mirror with a memory'. Today, we use the concept of the 'mirror' in talking about the relationship between digital culture and society, which can be accurate or disorienting (or both).

In the Victorian period, mirrors and cameras were part of a growing plethora of consumer culture that focused on appearance. Both technologies were and are used to scrutinize, assess, monitor and value the human face; both have their modern roots in the Renaissance, though their history stretches far back into antiquity; both produced results that were subject to ethical, moral and psychological judgements.

But whereas cameras are modern, mirrors have been around for hundreds, even thousands, of years, helping to tell us what we look like. This visual self-consciousness – cultivated through mirrors and later photography – has defined how we see ourselves, and each other. Why mirrors became commonplace, how they were made and used and what people did with them are essential parts of the modern story of facehood, as we will discover in the next chapter.

3.
Mirrored

> Fool, why try to catch a fleeting image, in vain? What you search for is nowhere: turning away, what you love is lost! What you perceive is the shadow of reflected form: nothing of you is in it. It comes and stays with you, and leaves with you, if you can leave!
>
> Ovid, *Metamorphoses*, 35–6

How many mirrors do you have in your home? Most people own at least one, propped up in the bathroom for shaving and cosmetic use; households with women are said to have more, including a full-length one for checking outfits – but surely that is an outdated view of gender and appearance? I own five: a full-length mirror I inherited from my daughter when she moved out; an Art Deco one in the front room bought from an antique shop for aesthetics rather than function; a small round, magnifying mirror that I keep in my make-up bag; a Moroccan silver one I was given for my thirtieth birthday and keep in the hall, for those last-minute checks before opening the front door; and one on the dressing table, with light bulbs around the edges, which I have never used because it didn't come with a proper plug.

I don't consider myself vain – having prosopagnosia, or face-blindness, helps with that – and it isn't unusual for other people in the Global North to have closer to ten or twelve mirrors in their homes. Such a casual inventory of mirrors marks an extraordinary change in our relationships with our reflection; until the Industrial Revolution, when mirrors became cheaper and mass-produced, most people didn't own even one mirror, let alone five.

How did they cope? Well, most people in the past didn't spend as much time looking at themselves, or worrying about their faces, as we do. Some rich people might have thought about it more; after all, mirrors themselves date back thousands of years, at least to 6000 BCE. But those mirrors were not just for looking in.

Throughout history, and today, especially in small, urban spaces, mirrors are used to reflect light and make homes seem larger and more aesthetically pleasing. Mirrors have also been used to turn images of the camera obscura the right way up; to see around corners in improvised military devices; to cast spells and divine the future; to repel evil spirits and even to communicate with the dead.

The Victorian belief that mirrors had some spiritual or supernatural function has a lengthy history across cultures: in the Jewish tradition, when mourning or sitting shiva, mirrors are covered when a person dies, allowing the bereaved to focus on their grief rather than earthly appearances; Islamic tradition holds that uncovered mirrors might invite jinn (spirits that could be evil) or negative spiritual influences into the home; Chinese and East Asian traditions cover mirrors in case they disrupt the soul's progress or invite evil spirits in; an ancient myth says that all mirrors are gateways to a parallel world, where the people we see are twisted and homicidal versions of ourselves. In 'William Wilson' and the other doppelgänger stories we encountered in the previous chapter, mirrors were a common plot device to reflect some psychic split.

The conceit that there is another person, or spirit, in the mirror – and that there might even be a whole other world inside it – is also commonplace in the Western tradition. As a child I used to sneak up on the bathroom mirror, certain that if I timed it right, the 'mirror me' would be caught unawares. From Lewis Carroll's *Through the Looking-Glass* (1871) to Naomi Klein's *Doppelganger: A Trip into the Mirror World* (2023), the idea of a mirror world has shifted from fantasy to digital reality; it is a common theme in horror films and ghost stories such as *Candyman* (1992). Even today I will not stand in front of a mirror and recite 'Candyman' five times in case I summon a man with a hook from his grave.

These cultural fears and fascinations reveal something profound about mirrors: they don't just show us our faces – they hint at an uncanny space between our inner and outer selves. They are a fertile space for the invention of all kinds of ideas about identity, and reality. It is only since the Victorian period, with the development of gas lighting, and a wide range of consumer goods focused on appearance, that we think of mirrors as principally things to see ourselves in.

It is perfectly acceptable to look at our own reflection today, and yet historically vanity has been frowned upon, or seen as narcissistic. Nowadays we use that term to describe a collection of personality traits characterized by selfish entitlement and callousness, and a lack of empathy that is pathological. But the origin of narcissism as a word and a concept lies in the Greek legend of Narcissus, a boy who fell in love with his own reflection in the water.

As described in 9 CE, in Book Three of Ovid's *Metamorphoses*, Narcissus was the son of the river god Cephissus and the water nymph Liriope. An exceptionally handsome youth, Narcissus was coldly indifferent to his admirers, including the mountain nymph Echo. By the time she fell in love with Narcissus, Echo had already been cursed by Zeus's wife Hera for distracting the goddess with her constant chatter. Hera's punishment was to take away Echo's voice: she could only ever repeat the last words spoken to her. When she was rejected by Narcissus, Echo pined away from heartbreak and died. All that remained was that sad echo, following travellers through caves and mountains.

Nemesis, the goddess of retribution and vengeance, punished Narcissus for his vanity and his indifference to Echo. Nemesis led Narcissus to a fountain, where he knelt to drink and, seeing his own reflection, fell madly in love with himself. Narcissus could not leave the object of his adoration, and remained by his reflection until he, like Echo, pined away. After his death, the flower that took his name – Narcissus (a pale, scented, daffodil-style member of the amaryllis family) – appeared by the fountain.

Mirrored

Picture Narcissus kneeling by that pool, transfixed by his own image. What did it mean to fall in love with your own reflection in a world where most people rarely saw themselves? This ancient myth feels remarkably contemporary in our age of selfies and social media, yet it emerged from a culture where encounters with one's own image were unusual.

The popularity of the tale of Narcissus peaked during the Renaissance, when ancient Greek and Roman texts were rediscovered, and humanism encouraged artists to revive classical values. Artists such as Caravaggio were also concerned with individualism and emotional experience. In his painting *Narcissus at the Fountain* (fig. 14), Caravaggio depicts Narcissus wearing an elegant brocade doublet, leaning forward as he stares enchanted at his reflection. The expression on Narcissus's face is one of open-mouthed curiosity, and the painting's composition – the upper half reflected in the lower

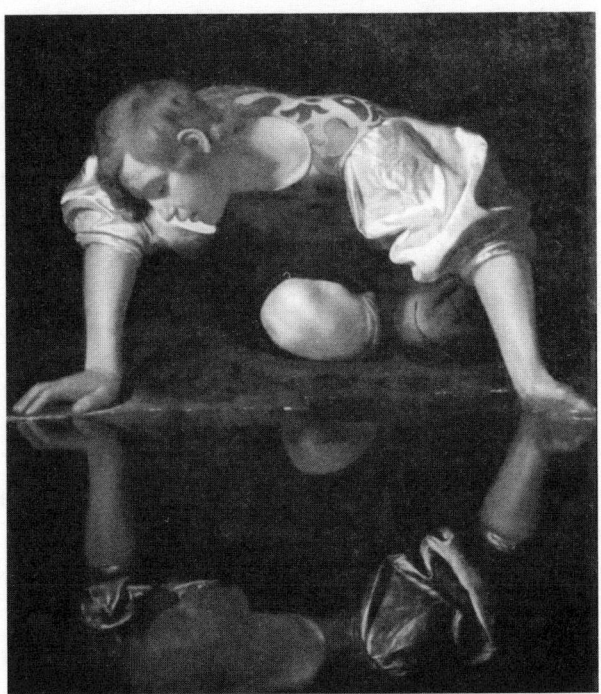

14. Caravaggio, *Narcissus at the Fountain*, 1597–99.

half – creates a circularity that reinforces the futile nature of Narcissus's self-love.

Artists in Caravaggio's time were increasingly interested in faces, using emotional expression to convey such moods as yearning and curiosity. Caravaggio employed mirrors and lenses to study his own reflection. He is believed to have used his own jaundiced reflection when painting his *Young Sick Bacchus* after recovering from hepatitis. Judging by the dramatic, almost photographic effects of his chiaroscuro (light and shadow), Caravaggio may well have been one of the first artists to use a camera obscura. Some researchers have even suggested his studio was a life-sized camera obscura, since he didn't make preparatory sketches. He may simply have employed mirrors and light to project images onto the studio walls.

If we think about Caravaggio staring into a mirror to accurately represent his face, we can imagine that his motive was different from Narcissus's adoring gaze at his own reflection. This was not an act of vanity, which according to the early Christian tradition was one of the Seven Deadly Sins. 'Your beauty should not come from outward adornment, such as elaborate hairstyles and the wearing of gold jewellery or fine clothes', as 1 Peter 3:3–4 cautioned. 'Rather it should be that of your inner self, the unfading beauty of a gentle and quiet spirit, which is of great worth in God's sight.' Of course, the beauty God wanted to see – that 'gentle and quiet spirit' – should also, according to physiognomy, be visible on the outside.

There is a preservation bias that means poorer people's lives often go undocumented (stone and precious metals surviving much longer than wood and leather). And most people in history did not wear gold jewellery and fine clothes; Peter was really admonishing the wealthy who had access to such things, as well as to mirrors. The average person would not have owned a mirror, or worn cosmetics, or routinely had their hair styled or dyed; nor would they have dressed in front of a mirror – why would most people bother, since they probably had one set of clothes that they wore day in, day out? And since they lived in places lit by candles or lamps, they had little opportunity to stare at their own faces after dusk, as we do, in unforgiving, artificial light.

Can you imagine navigating the world with such limited self-knowledge, where your own face was more of a mystery to yourself than to those around you?

As far back as the ancient world, however, those with enough wealth, status and reason to worry about their appearance certainly used mirrors – though they were made very differently from modern ones. As early as 3100 BCE, Egyptians fashioned mirrors out of polished bronze and copper, as well as the volcanic rock obsidian. Wealthy women rouged their lips and cheeks, stained their nails with henna and applied thick kohl, made from lead, copper, ash or burnt almonds, to their eyes and eyebrows. They probably had servants or slaves who would have assisted them to dress and prepare their faces, but the prevalence of obsidian mirrors suggests that, even so, wealthy women spent time admiring the results.

In the collections of the Metropolitan Museum of Art in New York there is an Egyptian mirror that dates from the second millenium BCE. Made of copper alloy rather than obsidian, the mirror was one of several found in the tomb of Hatnefer, a wealthy woman in her sixties who also had in her tomb a bronze razor and a cosmetic box. The handle of the mirror is decorated with the emblem of Hathor, the goddess of love, beauty and pleasure. In legend, Hathor possessed a magic mirror, which could see into the future.

As ceremonial, divinatory aids, mirrors allowed people to communicate with supernatural beings in other realms. For ancient Egyptians, the mirror could contain the 'ka', the life force or vital essence of a person, which survived death and could reside in statues and images. Mirrors would be wrapped up when not in use for this reason, ensuring that the door to the spirit world was closed. It is also why women like Hatnefer were buried with a mirror – it helped the souls of the deceased to recognize themselves in the afterlife.

The magical properties of mirrors did not die with the ancient Egyptians. In the fourteenth century CE, the Aztec divinity Tezcatlipoca owned an obsidian mirror that allowed him to see into the future, and into people's hearts – a kind of fortune-telling known as 'scrying'. In sixteenth-century England the occultist, mathematician and astrologer John Dee – referred to by Queen Elizabeth I as 'my philosopher' – picked up an Aztec obsidian mirror on his travels. He kept this black glass mirror in a sharkskin case, when he wasn't using it to 'peer into the future'. Dee's mirror, perfectly circular with a long handle, now resides in the British Museum.

Elizabeth's own mirrors, it is said, were hidden on her instruction as she aged, and she could not bear to look at herself. We don't know whether this is true – nor whether, as contemporaries reported, her ladies-in-waiting played a cruel trick on her by painting her nose red, knowing that she would never find out.

Because mirrors were beyond the reach of most people, we can only imagine that they saw themselves, in the main, as Narcissus had, in a watery reflection, or in some other shiny surface – a polished metal tool, perhaps (pewter, copper or bronze cooking equipment being for the wealthy).

What did it mean to an individual's sense of self, or self-consciousness, that they saw their face infrequently, if at all? Remember that this was also before the age of photography, so it is entirely reasonable to believe that a person might go from birth to death without seeing themselves at all, let alone with the regularity, frequency and detail we do in the modern West. There are still parts of the world today where mirrors are rare – especially within rural communities in the Global South.

Without mirrors, we must rely on the feel of our faces beneath the fingers and responses of other people, to determine whether our appearance is pleasing. We might also see ourselves in our loved one's eyes – in the reflection in their pupil; this is where the expression 'apple of my eye' comes from – in Old English the pupil was called the apple because it was round and shiny. The phrase also appears in the Bible ('keep me as the apple of the eye', Psalm 17:8), meaning that if you keep something that close, it must be precious to you.

Mirrored

What difference must it make to our awareness of our appearance and identity if our sense of self develops in relation to others, rather than to our own reflection? It must make us less self-conscious and self-critical; certainly that's what anthropologists found when comparing children's mirror behaviours in Kenya and Fiji with their counterparts in North America.

People living in fifteenth-century Leicester, an English market town, or Antwerp, a busy port in Belgium, for example, would not have been exposed to an endless stream of visual images of faces they were encouraged to emulate; no advertising, no photography, no promises of a better, happier you.

Might that absence of consumer messaging, in the fifteenth century, have represented a kind of psychological freedom, by today's standards?

Without constant visual reminders of how you looked, and how you didn't measure up, I wonder whether the face might have been experienced more as a tool for expression and communication than as an object for evaluation and improvement.

If we fast-forward from our fifteenth-century imaginaries to the seventeenth century, life for inhabitants of Leicester would have changed relatively little in terms of wealth and material goods; it would still be focused on local crafts and textile production. By contrast, Antwerp remained one of the largest cities in Europe, and a major centre of production for a range of expensive and fashionable consumer goods.

By the seventeenth century, Antwerp's merchant class would have been living in a much more 'modern' world than the Leicester gentry. Mirrors were everywhere – in the homes of the wealthy; in public buildings and churches; in the windows of glassmakers' shops; in barber-surgeons and apothecaries; and in taverns. Small, cheap mirrors would have been available for individuals to purchase, if they had enough money and desire. There would have been *some* mirrors in Leicester, but certainly not in the same numbers or of the quality as those found in Antwerp.

Mirrors became necessities in a world concerned with appearance and individualism, as demonstrated in chapter one by the growth of portraiture. The humanism that underpinned Renaissance art and led to an intense interest in the human face helped spread portraiture through the mercantile class – and drove the desire for material goods centred on appearance.

Technological developments helped both to meet and to feed the desire to see the face – this echoes the pattern we saw with the development of photography in the previous chapter, where growing public interest drove technical innovations, which in turn made the technology more accessible, and further increased demand. Similarly, increased demand for mirrors led to improvements in making and selling them.

The mirrors that met the needs of the market were no longer made from obsidian, as many were in the ancient world, but from glass, and the best results were pioneered by the Venetians.

Glass mirrors had existed in the medieval period, created by applying a layer of metal to glass. But the degree of heat needed to melt the metal, and the combined challenge of blowing glass, meant that mirrors tended to be small and convex. They were also rare – artists occasionally used them from the fifteenth century to explore perspective and composition, but the probable first use of a convex mirror in a home in any source is Jan van Eyck's *The Arnolfini Portrait* (fig. 15), in which the artist's presence is detectable in the glass.

The other best-known use of a convex mirror in art is probably Parmigianino's *Self-Portrait in a Convex Mirror* (fig. 16), which was painted nearly a century later. Outside of art, convex mirrors allowed bankers and moneylenders to survey an entire room immediately; as with other mirrors, they were also thought to have magical powers. In France convex mirrors were placed near doors and windows to ward off evil; the popular name for them was 'oeil de sorcière' ('witch's eye').

Mirror production wouldn't increase, or advance on the convex mirror, until the rest of Europe developed the skills that artisans had in Venice, specifically on the island of Murano, the centre of glassmaking since the thirteenth century. Murano glass was so

Mirrored

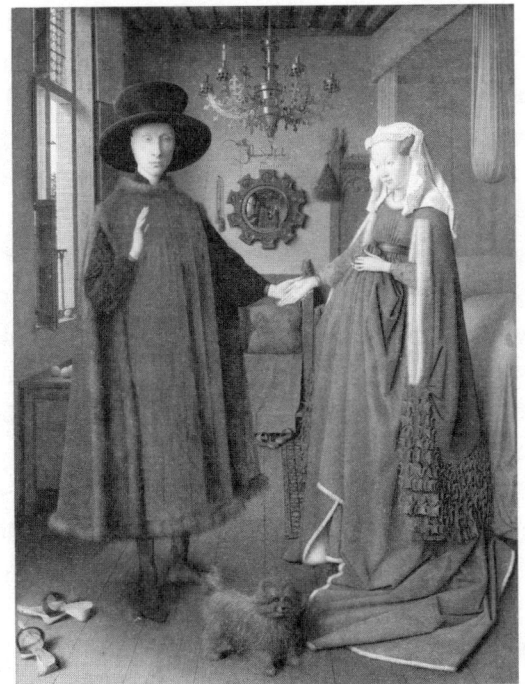

15. Jan van Eyck, *The Arnolfini Portrait*, 1434.

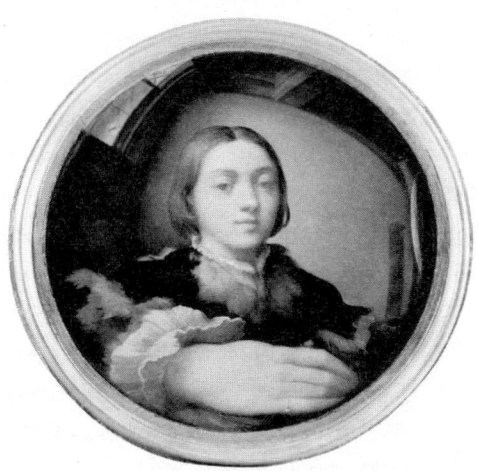

16. Parmigianino, *Self-Portrait in a Convex Mirror*, c. 1524.

important to Venice's tax income and international status that glassmakers were not permitted to leave the island or share the secrets of production. If a man escaped, he could be hunted down by an assassin. Glassmakers and their families were squirrelled away on an island sufficiently far outside the city to keep Venice safe (glass factories had a habit of burning down).

Since Venice started flourishing as a trading centre in the Middle Ages, dominating trade between Europe, North Africa and the Middle East, all kinds of treasures were bought and sold in the city: spices, jewels, silks, ivory and glass. Through its contacts, Venice also benefited from the influence of Syrian and Egyptian glassmaking, which was far more developed than in Europe.

In this tightly controlled world of glassmaking secrets, where knowledge was a matter of life and death, Murano mirror makers began to overlay glass with silver from the 1500s. This trick allowed much clearer reflections than those possible with the best obsidian or metal. These mirrors were rare and in great demand throughout the 1600s, until the French company Saint-Gobain lured a few artisans from Murano to Paris, where they perfected the method of casting large glass mirrors. The French then dominated mirror production in the seventeenth century, with glassmakers using mercury to add reflective coatings to glass – with no small impact on their health.

Who or what was driving this market for mirrors? In part, they continued to have spiritual significance, as well as being used in scientific experiments – even before Isaac Newton invented his reflecting telescope in 1668. And their importance in architecture and decorating grew with consumer culture; before the invention of gas lighting, the effects of sun and candlelight were enhanced by the clever positioning of mirrors.

One example is the Hall of Mirrors that was constructed between 1678 and 1684 in the French palace of Versailles. When built, the Hall was 73 metres long and boasted 357 mirrors; during daylight, the mirrors reflected the castle gardens in all seasons; during the evenings, they reflected candlelight, trebling the amount of light from each candle. The mirrors also conveyed the wealth and importance of Louis XIV and his successors, since mirrors were still luxury goods. Versailles was a coup for French mirror makers; the Hall of Mirrors was the first major commission that broke Venice's European monopoly.

I have noted the increasing use of mirrors as a status symbol, and the public demand for mirrors as linked to individualism and the face. We also need to recognize their prevalence as part of a more general self-consciousness about individual appearance and grooming. By the eighteenth century, people cared more about how they looked than they ever had before. It was necessary to look a certain way to thrive in wealthy or mannered society, and facial appearance, like habits and speech and gait, was governed by etiquette and fashion.

In other words, faces had to be managed in new ways – in the facial expressions that they wore (the subject of chapter six), as well as their grooming. Men were expected to be clean-shaven, with their eyebrows tamed, and men and women alike worried about their teeth and their smiles.

Razors were available for men to shave at home without traipsing to the barbers' salons; new designs of spectacles came out, with arms that reached around the head ('temple spectacles') or could slide inside the fibres of a wig ('wig spectacles'), as seen in Joshua Reynolds's *Self-Portrait* of circa 1788 (fig. 17). Spectacles became a symbol of intelligence for men in the reading salons and coffee houses of the eighteenth century; once only a sign of disability, they became evidence of learning and thought. Not so for women – in the main, beauty rather than intellect was expected to grace the face.

One exception to this rule was women's social use of the lorgnette, a pair of spectacles mounted on a handle, the precursor of modern opera glasses. The name lorgnette derives from the French word *lorgner*, meaning to 'ogle', or eye furtively. It was precisely this subtle and subterfuge dimension that inspired new designs, such as the 'jealousy lorgnette', which was constructed only for one eye to

The Face

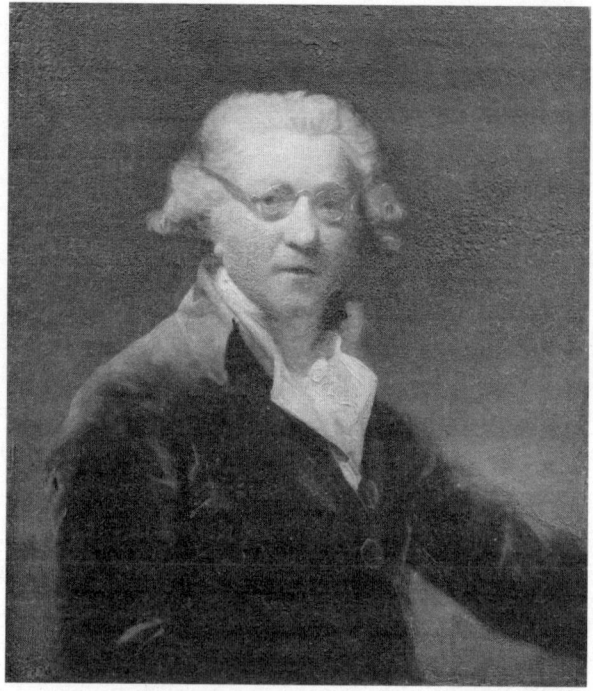

17. Joshua Reynolds, *Self-Portrait*, c. 1788.

peer through; the other contained a mirror so that the user could surreptitiously peer at people behind or alongside.

In the eighteenth century, famous users of the jealousy lorgnette included Jeanne Antoinette Poisson, Marquise de Pompadour (best known as Madame de Pompadour), who became the official mistress of Louis XV in 1745, and whom we shall shortly meet at her toilette.

Far more than a mere accessory, or aid to vision, the jealousy lorgnette provided a means for women to look at others without being discovered, and by the nineteenth century it had moved out of the theatre as a prop and into the fashionable wardrobe of most wealthy Europeans – and mostly women, as spectacles became more common for men.

We find a similarly gendered trend with facial cosmetics, which were once common in upper-class households of France and England, regardless of gender or age. Eyebrows were darkened and teeth brightened. Hairpieces and wigs were used to add volume to hair that was curled and brushed through with starch and powdered. The goal was a pale complexion – lead powder was used to whiten faces; rouge was applied to lips and cheeks. White face powder had been used since the Elizabethan period, commonly made from starch or lead, to emphasize the fact that wealthy white people didn't have to go outside and work in the fields in all weathers.

While it did not reflect modern forms of racism as defined by science in the Victorian period, pale skin was particularly linked with superiority, with European imperialism and colonization. Small black face patches, made from fabric or fur and developed in the Renaissance to cover scars and blemishes, were also in favour; sometimes these beauty spots or 'mouches' were used by the European aristocracy, and not only to cover up signs of smallpox, which was widespread across eighteenth-century Europe.

Mouches had increased in popularity during the reign of Louis XIV. Their shapes were infinite – moons, stars, hearts, ships – and they were kept in exquisite boxes made from gold or ivory or silver: *boîtes à mouche* ('fly boxes'). Such playful fashionable accoutrements made wealthy faces even more distinct from those of the peasantry, especially since they were used according to a secret code – a precursor of fan codes in the Victorian period, when the positioning of fans conveyed its own language of flirtation. A mouche on the right or left cheek in Britain could convey Tory or Whig sympathies; an engaged woman might wear a heart patch on her left cheek that she switched to her right after marriage; a mouche on the cheek indicated flirtatiousness, by the lower lip, discretion, and the corner of the eye: passion. Was this widespread? Probably not.

Yet when faces were not only a canvas to display beauty and expression, but a complex signalling device, the mirror was essential for checking your appearance, and for ensuring your face was sending exactly the right message.

We can see these fashions in eighteenth-century cosmetics, clothing and face adornments in the material culture of 'the toilette', which became a sociable event for the wealthy. At the centre of that toilette was a mirror, such as that received by the Duchesse de Cadaval, Henriette Julie Gabrielle de Lorraine – a prominent figure in the eighteenth century, known for her luxury and the quality of her belongings. An elaborate table mirror was commissioned for the duchesse in 1739, as part of a silver toilette set.

In such wealthy households, a maid would sponge-bathe and dress her mistress, who would spend hours getting her hair done, eating her breakfast from a tray, writing letters and entertaining friends. This made the toilette a semi-public as well as a private event. Rather like Johannes Gumpp's *Triple Self-Portrait* (fig. 18), in which we see the artist peering into the mirror on his left, while that same face appears on the easel to his right, the duchesse would have self-consciously put on her public face, simultaneously aware of others watching, and of the artifice involved.

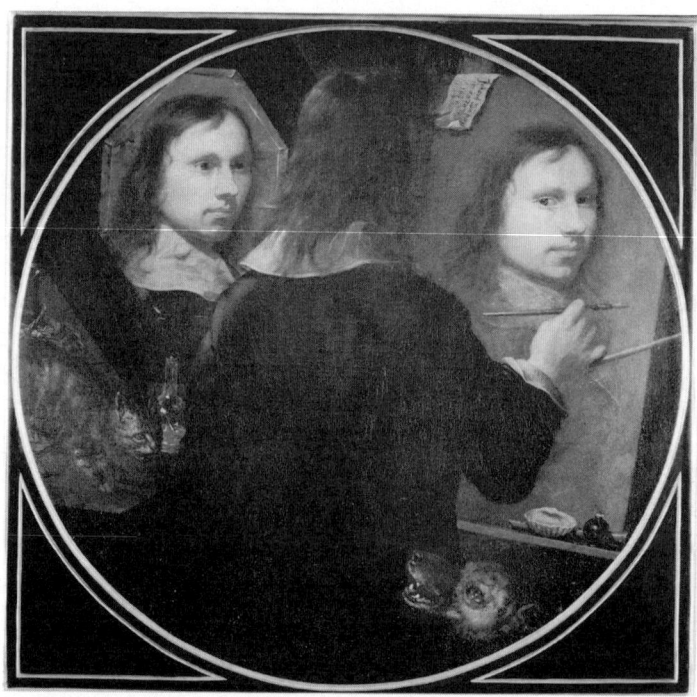

18. Johannes Gumpp, *Triple Self-Portrait*, 1646.

This layering of intimacy around the mirror is clear in François Boucher's painting *Pompadour at her Toilette* (1750) (fig. 19). One of many paintings commissioned of the subject, it depicts Madame de Pompadour, whose fondness for the lorgnette we saw earlier. In Boucher's painting the sitter is turned to the viewer, with her mirror visible to the right. She holds a brush with pink powder at its tip and is suspended in the act of applying rouge to her cheeks. The sitter's whiteness, beauty and youth are on display, within the context of the Rococo era's interest in soft palettes and aristocratic beauty. She is the artist as well as the sitter, busy curating the image she must present to the court to maintain her privileged position.

In eighteenth-century art, the mirror is often an intimate witness to this transformation from private self to public persona. And by the following century, cheaper mirrors became available for the middling sorts, and even some poorer people. As industrial

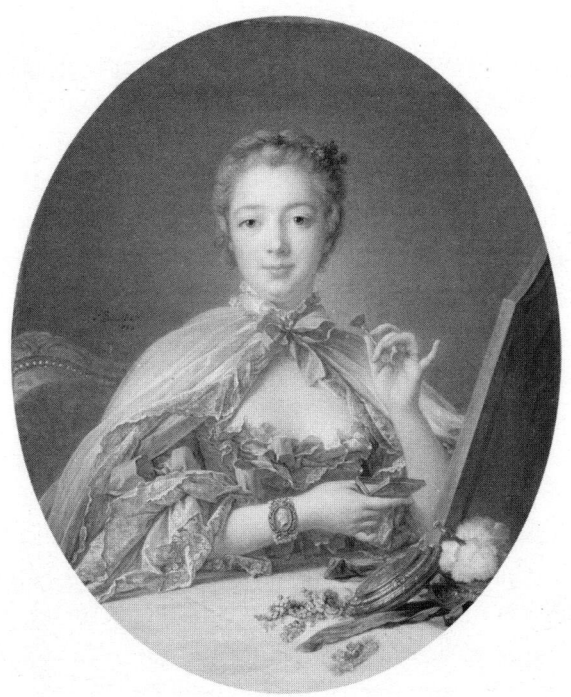

19. François Boucher, *Pompadour at Her Toilette*, 1750,

production expanded the market, women's periodicals such as the *Englishwoman's Domestic Magazine* urged readers to use not one but three mirrors, so that every surface and angle of their faces could be looked at. Since gas lighting exposed you to scrutiny in a way that candles didn't, you had always to be mindful of being watched. As Christina Rossetti wrote in her poem 'A Royal Princess' in 1851:

> All my walls are lost in mirrors, whereupon I trace
> Self to right hand, self to left hand, self in every place,
> Self-same solitary figure, self-same seeking face.

The idea of our appearance being constantly under scrutiny will be felt by many readers, and it is even truer of the twenty-first century than it was in the nineteenth. But it was changes in the material culture, attitudes and concerns of the Victorians that made possible our current obsession with the face – as an object of consumption and desire.

We have seen how for the Victorians the reinvigoration of classical beliefs, including physiognomy and an intense focus on racial and ethnic differences, reasserted the importance of whiteness and beauty. What could be seen, and classified, and compared, was very important in defining who and what mattered.

Mirrors, like light and photography, both symbolically and practically reinforced these hierarchical values. Shops and department stores used mirrors to entice customers in, to invite them to imagine how they would look in this necklace or that coat. Consumer goods, like the special objects on display in the newly established museums, were kept behind glass. Coveted items were theoretically available, but just out of reach.

This process invoked a democracy of desire, a trick of consumer consumption that gives the illusion of access. We can't all afford the things that would make us feel or look beautiful, though the clear glass makes it possible for us to imagine that we might; it is a levelling of yearning, not of possession. In *Theory of the Leisure Class* (1899) the American sociologist Thorstein Veblen referred to the industrial age as one of 'conspicuous consumption'; for the first time in history, and beyond the ranks of the nobility, there were people whose lives were not dedicated to work. Through leisure and shopping, they could define their identity, and show that they had taste, status and wealth.

And we do it too – we buy things in the often unconscious belief that we are buying not only the object but the lifestyle. This is the principle of consumer capitalism, which we see endlessly on social media; people scroll through Instagram, yearning to have what the Kardashians have, and believing it could be possible, if they bought a certain lipstick or had their belly fat moved to their cheeks.

In the mirror we see the problem and the solution; we see our flaws and we imagine how they might be fixed.

Now, the world of conspicuous consumption in the nineteenth century seems far removed from those Victorian photographers we met in the previous chapter – the ones who captured and compared human faces. But was it?

There were, in fact, some striking connections. And not just because fashion advertisers were using the same tool – photography – as the criminologists and anthropologists who sorted people into hierarchies from normal to deviant, civilized to primitive. They were all singing from the same song sheet.

What counted as desirable in fashion and advertising – whiteness, beauty, symmetry – were the same values that showed up in the sciences of race and crime. And those values didn't appear from nowhere; they were rooted in old ideas about reading faces and classical ideals but given a shiny new 'objective' veneer thanks to the new technologies of photography and the mirror: what you saw was what you got – or so it seemed.

For Victorian scientists, the whole world was a mirror, reflecting their presumptions about who belonged where. Sigmund Freud, in order to develop his theories of mind, famously analysed the behaviour of children his best-known case study being 'Little Hans', a boy who developed a fear of horses (which mattered in Freud's time more than it does today, since horse-drawn carriages were common on the streets of Vienna). Charles Darwin also studied children in order to understand human behaviour – specifically, he studied his own children as primitive humans, in much the same way that other scientists observed criminals, slaves and colonial subjects.

While Freud developed his theory of the Oedipus complex based on observations from children, Darwin watched the behaviour of his infant son, William Erasmus Darwin, during the 1840s to understand human evolution. How his son (affectionately called 'Doddy') behaved when he looked in the mirror was especially interesting to Darwin, particularly when he compared Doddy's responses with those of Jenny, an orangutan he had observed at the London Zoo in 1838.

'Three or four days ago [Doddy] smiled at himself in glass,' Darwin noted in his diary, when Doddy was just five months old. Darwin was yet to publish *On the Origin of Species*, and he was still working out the relationship between humans and apes.

'How does [Doddy] know his reflection is that of [a] human being?' Darwin wondered. 'That he smiles with this idea, I feel pretty sure – Smiled at my image & seemed surprised at my voice coming from behind him, my image being in front.' By September of the same year, Doddy would turn and look at himself in the mirror when asked, 'Where is Doddy?' By the time he was one year old, he would kiss his reflection in the mirror. Doddy also recognized his own reflection in the pupil of his father's eye.

In comparing boy and orangutan, Darwin recalled how Jenny had seemed angry when teased over an apple by her keeper. How conscious was she of being an orangutan, he wondered; could she, like Doddy, be aware of her own existence? What did it mean to be conscious of one's own existence anyway?

These kinds of questions had been asked by scientists for hundreds of years; the belief that animals did not have consciousness, or a soul, was why vivisectionists had no qualms about dissecting them alive. The animal had no sense of pain, they reasoned, no consciousness. And yet, when Darwin held the mirror up to Jenny and her companion orangutan, he saw that:

> '... both were astonished beyond measure at looking glass, looked at it every way, sideways, & with most steady surprise. – after some time stuck out lips, like kissing, to glass ... at last put hand behind glass at various distances, looked over it, rubbed front of glass, made faces at it – examined whole glass – put face quite close & pressed it – at last half refused to look at it – startled & seemed almost frightened, & evidently became cross because it could not understand puzzle.'

So, the difference between humans and apes when it came to mirrors, as later experiments confirmed, was that humans would be transfixed and not lose interest, whereas apes became frustrated or bored. This observation helped Darwin determine that there was a hierarchy of mind between humans and apes – that the difference was one of degree rather than kind. It may not seem much to us, but it helped shape Darwin's theory of a shared ancestry between humans and other primates.

There have been other 'mirror tests' since, delving into the differences between humans and animals. When do animals recognize themselves? asked Gordon Gallup Jr, an American evolutionary psychologist, in 1970. To find out, he anaesthetized several different animals, before marking them with paint on an area of the body they could only see in the mirror – usually the forehead. When awake, the animal was shown its reflection in a mirror. If the animal recognized itself, it might rub at the mark on its forehead to try to remove it.

Not all species pass the Gallup test; great apes and elephants seem to recognize their own faces, as do manta rays, magpies, dolphins and some crabs. Dogs do not. And nor do most monkeys, pandas and sea lions. Yet dogs' faces are believed to have evolved in conjunction with human faces. It is likely that the 'puppy dog' expression, characterized by sad eyes and a crumpled brow, resulted from the co-evolution of a muscle between the eyes in dogs that was deliberately designed to get attention from humans.

That theory seems credible, given that dogs were first domesticated some 23,000 years ago in Siberia. To suggest that a dog has a less sophisticated sense of 'self' than a crab seems a stretch, which should alert us to the limits of such studies. The mirror test relies solely on visual recognition and doesn't consider species-specific or context-based reactions; nor does it include forms of self-recognition that aren't visual (like smell), and there are many – as we will find out in chapter eight.

The mirror clearly tells us something about being human – and what matters to us as social beings, as well as self-regarding ones. At the same time as a growing number of conduct books and behaviour guides were published, accompanying urbanization, increased consumerism and a rising middle class that wanted to know how to behave 'properly', the term 'mirroring' became popular from the 1800s, when new psychological theories came into being.

The themes of mimicry and imitation were popular for early psychologists – largely because of Darwin's work on mimicry in nature in *On the Origin of Species*; in his *The Expression of the Emotions* (1872) he also suggested that people might imitate displays of emotion to foster social bonding and communication.

By the twentieth century, the study of mirroring became more pronounced with social psychology and attachment theorists, and with the study of non-verbal communication – body language, gestures and facial expressions. The discovery of mirror neurons in the brain in the 1990s went further, showing a biological basis for human mimicry.

I am reminded of both my children, when they were about two years old, pulling faces at themselves in the mirror – faces that they had seen on the adults around them. They were learning how to emote, how to enter the world of the fully human, with expressions that were over the top admittedly – exaggerated caricatures of grief and delight – but important aspects of human communication for their social repertoire.

Our mirroring of the emotional expressions of others is normally more subtle – people often unconsciously settle into the rhythm of another person's body language, tone of voice and emotional expression, especially when conveying empathy.

When we spend time with people we like or admire, we might take this mirroring further, unconsciously copying their hairstyle or clothing, their verbal tics and even their values. In the 1950s, the American sociologists Paul Lazarsfeld and Robert Merton called this process homophily, meaning 'love of sameness'. It explains why humans often tend to form relationships with people who have similar backgrounds and experiences; they become symbolic mirrors in ways that bolster our self-esteem. We might even seek out friends whose faces resemble our own, much as some people subconsciously seek out romantic partners with similar facial structures.

Not all of us use our mirrors as a tool for conformity; for every push there is a pull, for every culture a counterculture. Sometimes, recreating and reimagining what we see in the mirror is a powerful act.

This is the case with Isabel Adomakoh-Young, the actor, drag king, writer and co-founder of Pecs: The All-Female and Non-Binary Drag Collective; for them, transforming into a man 'tunes me into a part of myself'. When a strikingly beautiful person applies facial hair, thickens up their eyebrows, contours their nose, and appropriates the expressions and mannerisms of a confident man, it forces you to think about the presumptions we make about a person's appearance – and the values we attach to that.

We tend not to think about the ways in which masculinity is as artificial as femininity in relation to faces and bodies; stereotypical feminine add-ons, such as long eyelashes and heels, are somehow recognized as additions, whereas cultivating a swagger or a stubbled chin are seen as naturally masculine.

The drag-king phenomenon reminds us that gender is a work in progress, and that what masculinity and femininity mean is always open to question. Think back to those eighteenth-century men with their white face paint and mouches. That was a declaration of status and class on the part of the aristocracy. Some middle-class men who emulated the wealthy wore make-up too, when they felt sufficiently confident about elevating their social status. They certainly weren't accused of being unmanly, or homosexual.

By the 1800s, men wearing make-up was no longer respectable. In France, it was condemned after the French Revolution, since it was associated with the aristocracy and moral corruption. In the United Kingdom, and more generally in Europe, a so-called 'Great Male' Renunciation' took place in the 1790s. The phrase was coined by the British experimental psychologist and psychoanalyst John Flügel to describe how respectable men stopped using cosmetics and bright fabrics and left such perceived frippery to women. Being useful rather than beautiful was what mattered for men; gone were the high heels, wigs and the tight-fitting breeches, and in came sombre dark suits and pantaloons. These changes coincided with the philosophical idea that men were rational, useful beings, whereas women were decorative beings and emotionally fragile.

It is telling that from the 1960s, when many post-war values were rejected, a sartorial revolution again took place. The decade was marked by a shift towards more flamboyant, colourful and experimental clothing; from the late 1970s to early 1980s, the New Romantics wore heavy make-up, and challenged traditional gender norms. Before Adam Ant, who could have predicted that white face paint and the mouche would be back in fashion?

Cosmetics and clothes have an element of play. For many people, changing their face with cosmetics, or filters, is enough. For others, a more permanent change feels necessary; for them the pursuit of a 'better' face is not only an opportunity but also an obligation in the pursuit of wealth, success and status.

That is the dark side of our life with mirrors; if we lack healthy self-esteem, we might seek it in the mirror, which can only tell us, like the magic mirror in *Snow White*, that there is someone far more beautiful. Some of us develop an unhealthy obsession with our own flaws – Body Dysmorphia Disorder (BDD) was recognized as a rare psychological pathology in the 1980s; its prevalence has risen with the visual social media of the 2010s.

Social media has been called a mirror with a memory – the same name originally given to the camera. Today, many cannot separate their fixation with the mirror in the bedroom from the mirror of the internet. Several mental-health disorders are marked by staring, disconsolately, into the mirror – not only BDD but also Narcissistic Personality Disorder (NPD), Obsessive-Compulsive Disorder (OCD), Eating Disorders (ED), and more general forms of depression and anxiety.

Whether or not it becomes pathological, increasing numbers of people are dissatisfied with their faces – even more than their bodies. In part this is because we can cover up our bodies easier than we can our faces; but it's also because our faces are judged, critiqued and used as the focus of all our social interactions.

Why are so many of us obsessed with what we see in the mirror? Because what we see there is never just a face – it is a canvas onto which we project centuries of accumulated meanings about beauty, identity, worth and power.

Surrounded by mirrors – literal, symbolic, digital – we have internalized those meanings and made the face a commodity, a thing external to us that must be maintained and improved in the quest for love, wealth and status. Just as post-industrial bodies became machines to be fuelled and pushed to their breaking point – no pain, no gain! – our faces have become projects to be perfected. We work on them the way we might work on assembly lines, with the same relentless efficiency, the same fear of obsolescence.

Modern consumerism doesn't just sell us products; it sells the imperative to never stop looking, never stop improving, never be enough. Our smartphones are the magic mirrors in our pocket that give us a thousand daily verdicts on how we fall short. We have made the most intimate part of ourselves – the face that our friends recognize, our lovers touch – into something that must earn its worth in the marketplace of attention. The very thing that is supposed to be *us* has become something we must endlessly strive to become. No wonder so many people end up feeling depressed and unworthy, victims of the Compare and Despair cycle.

The mirror has been at the heart of these psychological and social transformations – from a tool for communicating with the gods to a device for perpetual self-surveillance.

Some people feel the effects of that surveillance more profoundly than others. Our sense of self shifts during our lives, as does our willingness to buy into trends. It seems that Generation Z (generally meaning people born between 1997 and 2012) look in the mirror far more often than Generation X (those born between 1965 and 1980). City, University of London found that 90 per cent of girls aged 11–21 use filters when taking photos to alter skin tone, teeth, or facial structure, with negative effects on self-image.

Which brings us back to poor Narcissus. Unlike Narcissus, most of us do not stare adoringly at our reflections, but critically; we think we look too old, too fat, too saggy, too pale, too dark, too tired; that our noses are too big or our cheeks too large; our foreheads too wide or not wide enough.

Personally, I am conscious of my glabella, that area of the forehead between the eyebrows and just above the nose, which as you age, presents you with two deep '11' lines. Look in the mirror and frown – you will see what I mean. Women worry about such things more than men, often from necessity – men's frown lines mean they are considered authoritative; women's that they have 'resting bitch face'.

We are rightly more attuned to the nuances of gender than we once were, and you can't be a historian of the body without knowing how conditional sexed identity has always been. But when we look at the history of the face, we are also looking at the patriarchy.

When Victorian scientists invented human hierarchies, the top of the pyramid was not only white, but male. Across the world men still dominate the social structures, legal systems and cultural norms that dictate how we live; women have less access to formal power systems, leadership roles, economic opportunities and decision-making.

Women are also judged by their faces, and through internalized misogyny, all too often criticize other women for how they look. And probably because women have long been more closely judged by appearance, surveys suggest they still check mirrors more often – often twenty to forty times a day, compared with fifteen to thirty for men. What they focus on also differs; women tend to scrutinize flaws, especially online, while men look more lightly or admiringly.

This is changing as beauty standards shift – there is increasing expectation for men to look a certain way – but women are far from achieving parity. As the art critic John Berger put it in *Ways of Seeing*:

> Men act, and women appear. Men look at women. Women watch themselves being looked at. This determines not only most relations between men and women but also the relation of women to themselves. The surveyor of woman in herself is male: the surveyed is female. Thus, she turns herself into an object of vision: a sight.

Since the 1950s, women who are profoundly unhappy with that sight have had the option of another technological innovation, cosmetic surgery. Is this an extension to the beauty industry, with its plumping creams and whitening powders, or something else? Why shouldn't we upgrade and enhance and modify our faces, as we would our cars, houses and wardrobes, if a more beautiful face brings a happier existence and a better life? That is the argument of the cosmetic-surgery industry, after all.

But is it true? Does changing what we see in the mirror transform our lives for the better? What if making the face a commodity is a mistake – and what we are chasing a mere reflection? Let's turn to the next chapter and find out.

4.

Perfected

In June 2024, @estemedistanbultr, an Instagram account for the Este Medical Group in Turkey, which specializes in plastic surgery, dental work and hair transplants, posted a dramatic makeover to their 600,000 Instagram followers. It showed the face of a man who had undergone rejuvenation treatment, and the before-and-after photographs were striking. In the after image, Michael looked decades younger and more conventionally handsome with more hair, a slimmer, more angular face, no bags under the eyes, and a narrower nose.

How had this been achieved? According to the clinic: a facelift; a neck lift; the removal of fat from the upper and lower eyelids (blepharoplasty); face sculpting below the cheekbones (buccal fat removal); a nose job (rhinoplasty); and a hair transplant. The post went viral and was followed immediately by another series of transformations, this time showing one Miss Dilek, who had similarly been reshaped by a nose job, a facelift and fat removal. That post gathered more than 26,500 likes in two days.

Turkey has become a cosmetic-surgery hotspot, and many people who saw the post were staggered; 'This is virtually unbelievable, excuse me while I book my flight' was a typical response. Others were more sceptical: 'Is this legit or are we all getting trolled?'

Wondering whether the post was made by trolls or scammers is entirely reasonable, given how prevalent AI is becoming online and in advertising, and the parallel rise in online phishing scams. We live, increasingly, in a state of cognitive dissonance, where the lines of real and fake are blurred. Isn't it tempting to believe that such a visible transformation is possible, and attainable, especially at moments when we feel fat or old and irrelevant?

Why are so many of us willing to suspend disbelief? The answer lies in something we've encountered throughout this book: our deep-seated belief that attractive individuals are not just happier but *better* – more intelligent, more honest, more caring, more trustworthy, according to numerous surveys.

These theories, established by classical physiognomy and reinforced by nineteenth-century scientists, are powerful. No matter how much evidence there is to the contrary – the convicted killers Jodi Arias, Richard Ramirez and Ted Bundy all received media attention for their 'deadly' good looks.

No wonder plastic-surgery rates are rising. In 2018, the American Society of Plastic Surgeons estimated that $16.5 billion a year was spent on cosmetic enhancements, rising to $26 billion by 2022. Beauty tutorials received 169 billion YouTube views in 2018, and 50 per cent more by 2020. Some of this increase was exacerbated by lockdowns; people spent days staring at their own faces in video meetings, fantasizing about improving their homes, their bodies, their faces; and evenings watching the videos that promise to bring those improvements about. 'Zoom neck' emerged as a phenomenon and triggered a rush on requests for skin tightening.

We do not ordinarily stare at our own faces when we are speaking to other people, so the pandemic gave a unique opportunity for fretting about saggy jowls, flat cheeks, wrinkles and neck skin. Personally, I have found that switching off the self-view on Zoom or Teams allows us to focus on the other person, as we would in real life, rather than on our own insecurities and perceived aesthetic shortcomings.

Remember our discussion of mirrors and how they changed our relationship with our own faces? The pandemic turned our screens into mirrors that we couldn't escape. Not only did those screens reflect an unsettling reality – they inundated us with advertisements promising that a solution was just a scalpel away.

What people want to achieve with surgery varies. Young people are more likely to seek perfection; as we age, our desire shifts slightly – we are more likely to want to have the face and body we had at twenty or thirty or before we had children. In both cases the presumption is that there is value – emotional, financial, social, sexual and economic – in looking a certain way – the idea that beauty correlates with success is enshrined in culture, advertising, marketing and books with titles like *Beauty Pays: Why Attractive People Are More Successful* (2011) by the economist Daniel Hamermesh.

Before social media, if we thought about cosmetic treatments, we had to book a visit to a clinic to talk about options and get a quote. That required a series of conscious and physical steps, a degree of planning, time and thought. Today, we can lie in bed in the early hours scrolling through our phones and accidentally come across a reel that offers us a better face. We still need to make the journey to a clinic, but we can put a nose job or a facelift into our metaphorical shopping basket.

Cosmetic surgeons use Instagram, TikTok and other platforms precisely because they are visual, and they align neatly with the idea of before-and-after that is well established in our cultural imagination. Myths and fairy tales were full of Cinderella-style transformations long before rom-coms, weight-loss advertisements and home makeovers. A frog becoming a prince or a servant girl a princess suggests a world in which we can be seen 'as we really are' or how we want to be seen – a carriage instead of a pumpkin, a footman instead of a mouse.

We are all prone to do it but focusing on the before-and-after also promises an accessible and simple act. We enlist builders to transform our kitchens, not thinking about the inevitable weeks of waiting and delays and additional costs. Similarly – and with much more significant consequences – we might obsess over Kris Jenner's deep-plane facelift, which as I write has just gone viral, without thinking about the raw realities of surgery. We put to the back of our minds the bruising, swelling, pain, possible infection, as well as any potential negative feelings, such as shame, regret, embarrassment and disappointment. We ignore the fact that we might not like the result, or that looking thirty-five again might not fix our lives.

What we find on digital platforms is mostly unverified, and there is little regulation around what clinics can promise. This includes what outcomes can be achieved, practically, for a changed face, and emotionally, in terms of how much happier and more successful in love, life, work, we might be if only our nose wasn't so large, or our eyes so droopy. And haven't we all, at least once, thought maybe if . . . ?

I have, and more than once. In my mid-thirties, I visited a clinic in London for research; it was soon after a flurry of buy-one-get-one-free, mother-and-daughter cosmetic-surgery bargains offered by surgeons had been criticized by medical ethicists. Nobody seemed to be talking about the emotional power imbalance between the surgeon and the prospective patient, or the psychological effects of salespeople without any medical training wearing white coats. And I wanted to know what that felt like. Emboldened by a crusade for truth, I stripped off in front of the surgeon (who, incidentally, had undergone so much surgery herself that her face was distinctly feline). Then I asked her: 'OK, what would you do, if you were given free rein?'

It is not a question I would ask today. I am still interested in the answer, in an abstract, intellectual sort of a way, but fifteen years later, my skin isn't thick enough to hear it. On that afternoon in 2010, the surgeon inspected my face and body with practised, distanced, gloved hands. As she cast her expert eye over me, I felt removed from my body, as if I were a broken shoe and she, a cobbler, was readying to fix the heel.

Then I dressed while the surgeon took several thick albums of before-and-after photographs down from her shelves (this was the year that Instagram came out; digital photography existed but selfies wouldn't be widespread until 2012). Together we flicked through the albums, as if we were friends sharing holiday snaps. I could have a slimmer nose, like that woman; a chin tuck like that one; silicone implants in my cheeks, maybe, a brow lift, Botox? If I wanted body procedures too – fat taken from my thighs and added to my breasts, liposuction on my belly – I was looking at £17,000, as I told my friend over a stiff drink that evening – for results that would last ten years, tops, less time in the case of fat transfer.

If I were to take my insecurities to a similar clinic in 2025, I would be met with an even longer menu of options. I could resurface my skin with a laser, have my skin tightened using electromechanical devices; I could graft fat from anywhere on my body to plump up my cheeks; I could freeze the fat in my cheeks to slim them down; I could fill and flip my lips to make them poutier, I could get dental implants for a polar white smile, I could have the skin at the side of my eyebrow stretched out to create 'fox eyes'. The list goes on and on. I could, if I had a couple of years and £50,000 to spare, look like Miss Dilek. Or maybe even Michael.

The problem is that the figures known as Michael and Miss Dilek appear not to exist as presented on Instagram.

When the posts of @estemedistanbultr went viral, the British tabloid the *Daily Mail* interviewed several plastic and cosmetic surgeons to ask them whether these before-and-after images could really be the same people? The sugeons interviewed said no. Nigel Mercer, a plastic surgeon in Bristol, noted that Michael's eyebrow shape is 'completely different . . . [and] his face is a completely different shape, and I can't believe you can do that with just buccal fat removal'. Others agreed, saying that even if it were possible, then it would take many more operations than the clinics admitted to. And where were the scars?

The surgeons were even less convinced by Miss Dilek. They noted how different the skin tone and quality were on the images; the eyes were different colours. Bizarrely, I didn't notice this; the fact that I have prosopagnosia, or face-blindness, might have had a role in that – as we will see in chapter eight. But there is a more general, psychological reason why people might not observe such details: confirmation bias. We are culturally conditioned to think the before-and-after means a transition to something 'better' and less likely to notice clues that something doesn't fit.

Soon after the furore in the British tabloids, the Turkish TV channel Ekol TV tracked down the man in the after image. That person, whom I will call Mehmet, said, 'I am not the person in this news. I did not have a face transplant.' He had undergone a different surgery to his nose four years ago, which is presumably how the clinic had access to his photograph. Mehmet said that he would be taking legal action, as he was being harassed constantly: 'My phones have not stopped ringing. Messages keep coming in. I am tired.'

Why show such images? Well, it is effective clickbait: creating an image for impact takes people to the Instagram page and to the website where people can check prices, compare procedures and book themselves in. In the main there are no negative consequences for clinics that give misleading information.

And there is little effective legislation: cosmetic surgery is regulated by the Care Quality Commission in England, and the Food and Drug Administration in the U.S., and other countries have their own standards, but medical tourism means clinical practice can fall through the net.

Also, many forms of cosmetic intervention, for example Botox and fillers, have been poorly regulated in some countries, including the UK. In August 2025, the UK government announced new legislation to license cosmetic procedures and restrict the most invasive treatments to qualified healthcare professionals. The measures aim to protect the public from unsafe or unethical practices, but many details, including enforcement and who qualifies to operate, are still being developed.

It isn't unusual for patients, framed as 'customers' in the consumerist age of healthcare, to find themselves without recourse if treatments are unsatisfactory. And it's not good for nationally funded healthcare systems such as the National Health Service in England; when patients are back home with post-surgical crises, such as infections or necrosis, they end up carrying the can. So public-health systems deal with the challenges of surgeries that are private and for profit, while the patients/consumers are taking the risks. There are brilliant cosmetic surgeons out there who care deeply about their patients, but there are also many opportunistic surgeons who seem to be making hay while the sun shines.

Is it new to think about the face, or the body, this way – as something to be traded? Not entirely; historically, many people have been treated as commodities: slaves, sex workers, serfs, spouses. In the medieval and early modern economies, there was some obligation of care due from those in charge; less so in modern systems where we trade our industry – produced by our bodies – for a wage.

In many ways our emotions are also traded; we smile to keep our jobs, our reputations, our lives. Every day we all trade emotional expressions to smooth the wheels of social interaction. But it was with the emergence of capitalist consumer culture in the West that this idea became increasingly explicit and entangled with beliefs about face value.

By the late nineteenth century, shops and department stores were extending a variety of goods down the social chain. It was not only the rich who could afford material objects such as mirrors and razors and cosmetics and toiletries. Retailing was being turned over to the hands of corporate giants rather than individual shopkeepers in the U.S. and the U.K.; they had access to investment bankers and factory assembly lines that produced more goods in greater numbers than ever before.

The more people consumed, and what they consumed, became linked to their social identity and their sense of self in the world – and it was all underpinned by more and more emphasis on the idea of individualism that originated in the Renaissance. To keep the wheels of the consumer economy turning, people needed to be simultaneously filled with both desire and discontent.

'Keep the consumer dissatisfied' was how Charles Kettering, the director of the General Motors Research Laboratory, put it. 'It's a question of change, change all the time – and it's always been that way because the world only goes along one road, the road of progress.'

So, progress meant the constant creation of new needs and desires, and the simultaneous dissatisfaction with what we possess.

It is a road that brought us to both the climate disaster, and, I believe, the current mental-health crises in the West of loneliness, anxiety and depression. Because no matter what consumerism tells us, material things will never bring us what we crave: human connection and a sense of belonging.

Faces lie at the heart of our shared humanity. A fleeting glance that sparks recognition, eyes that light up with laughter or tenderness, the gentle curve of a smile shared over a meal, the warmth of a palm pressed against a beloved's cheek – our faces are the canvas of intimacy and understanding, instruments of communion, not commodities for consumption.

So how did we arrive at this moment, where the essence of our connection has become judged purely in aesthetic terms, as an object to be enhanced, traded and improved?

After the Depression, the Second World War, and its years of rationing, corporate advertisers stepped hard on the gas of progress. News media and television did this in increasingly visual ways, with advertising agencies invested heavily in professional photography to create eye-catching campaigns. For the first time, the face itself became a mass-produced object of desire, and not only in advertising. In cinemas, sirens of the silver screen – Judy Garland, Audrey Hepburn, Marilyn Monroe – specialized in the close-up, their trembling lips and shimmering eyes inviting viewers to emote, to feel, to desire.

Cinema encouraged new trends in face and body image as much as it promoted cigarette brands and designer clothing. This was a heyday for beauty salons, manicurists and hairdressers, as the cult of the body beautiful exploded across the U.K. and the U.S. And the same kinds of concerns were expressed about the societal effects of cinema and advertising on the minds of young, impressionable people that we see with social media (one difference, of course, being that cinema and advertising could not follow them *everywhere*).

Lipstick and hair rollers could only do so much. But by the 1950s, a new solution for those who wanted to look their best was becoming mainstream: cosmetic surgery – which took centre stage through a combination of consumer desire (subtly transformed into 'need'), surgical skills and the technology to make it possible.

Plastic surgery as a specialism dates back as far as Sushruta, the so-called 'father of surgery', in ancient India; the word 'plastic' comes from the Greek *plassein*, or 'to mould'. The earliest plastic surgeons were principally repairers of injury and disease. It is much more recent that the aesthetic notion of enhancement became a distinct subfield, though sometimes 'plastic' and 'cosmetic' are used interchangeably. I'm interested here in cosmetic or aesthetic surgery, and how that developed out of plastics.

Sushruta specialized in moulding new noses for those cut off as punishment (the routineness of which we saw in our discussion of portraiture). By the first century BCE, the Romans were undertaking surgical procedures, such as breast reduction, as well as fixing some of the noses that were hacked off in punishment, as we saw in chapter one.

There has always been an element of the aesthetic in plastic surgery. Since plastic surgeons operate on visible areas of the body, they have a pride in the visual that is not shared by orthopaedic surgeons, since bones are hidden. And sometimes that means that plastic surgeons' subjective view on beauty finds its way into the operating theatre; I have lost count of the number of women I have interviewed who were persuaded up a cup size by surgeons who believed that bigger was better. I have also heard stories of women undergoing mastectomies for cancer and saying they didn't want implants, only for their male surgeons to leave the empty breast behind, in case women 'changed their minds', or their husbands had an opinion.

Even allowing for the importance of the aesthetic in plastic surgery, there is a difference between healing faces that have been damaged and changing faces that are otherwise healthy. A few distinct circumstances had to come together for purely aesthetic surgery to become skilful, as well as viable and desirable.

The precipitating event for such a skill was the First World War.

There is nothing like war for creating opportunities for medical experimentation – and in the First World War, surgeons learned to work quickly, developing new techniques to treat a huge amount of injuries. The combination of heavy-duty ballistics and trench warfare were a terrible combination for a young man's face. The weapons of war – high-explosive shells, machine guns, poison gas – created casualties who needed rehabilitative surgery, skin grafts, limb repair.

Portraits of the surgeons who established modern plastic surgery – especially Harold Gillies in the First World War and Archibald McIndoe in the Second – line the walls of many a plastic surgeon's office; they are a nod to surgical lineage. But when the wars ended, there were no more soldiers to fix. Here was a specialism trained in repairing faces that now had no faces to repair – no market. But they soon found one: in post-war consumerism, and among women bedazzled by constant projections of beauty, who wanted – or felt they somehow ought to have – the faces (and perhaps lives) of society belles, models and screen goddesses.

Were a willing market, surgeons' skills and silicone enough to launch cosmetic or aesthetic surgery as a proper field? No – there also had to be a clinical need. Traditionally, the Hippocratic Oath and, later, the Nuremberg Code of 1947 affirmed that informed and voluntary consent was essential to medical ethics.

How do we assess whether a patient's psychological need is sufficiently pressing to justify medical risks? In addressing this question, medical consumerism found powerful allies in the newly emergent specialisms of psychology and psychiatry.

The first silicone breast enlargement became possible in 1962, when new medical-grade silicone made such procedures technically feasible. Around the same time, small-breastedness was newly framed as a source of psychological distress, linking for the first time small-breastedness ('hypomastia'), depression, and low self-worth. The 'inferiority complex', developed by Alfred Adler and Sigmund Freud, offered another rationale for cosmetic treatment.

If healthy psychological development required individuals to feel confident about their appearance, and if low self-esteem represented a genuine mental-health concern, then cosmetic surgery became not merely desirable but essential. This reframing aligned perfectly with the expectations of consumer culture, particularly in the U.S. – if you don't like something, fix it.

Meanwhile, beauty standards have shifted like trends in any consumer market. In the 1920s, fashionable female faces featured pale skin and small mouths; by the 1950s, fuller lips and figures had become desirable. The 1960s saw a curious contradiction: whereas breasts were flattened to achieve a boyish silhouette, eyes were dramatically enlarged with make-up to create a saucer-like effect. Even as women gained greater political and economic rights during this era, the prevailing feminine ideal emphasized a girlish, sexually available and passively childlike appearance.

In the 1970s, many women opted for a more natural appearance, eschewing make-up and keeping their body hair; by the 1990s the third wave of feminism saw a snap back again, with 'girl power' being all about make-up and beauty, and championing the idea that women could be empowered and wear high heels, because power was associated with women using sexuality to their own advantage. Brows made it big in the 2000s, and the false-eyelash/enormous blow-up-doll mouth combination – lifted directly from pornography – became ubiquitous during the 2010s and 2020s. One could write a whole book about these changes, and how they reflect gender politics and threats to patriarchy.

Peer pressure has been behind consumer capitalism since its conception. All those eighteenth-century men and women buying exotic teas and silver teapots were motivated by an element of the same 'fear of missing out' that we have today (though we have the acronym to express its modern, heightened, turbo-charged, industrialized importance: FOMO).

It isn't just the desire for the new that keeps the plates of capitalism spinning; it's also the threat of failure. What one doesn't possess is as much an indicator of status as what one does.

It is a simple fact that people who are not regarded as beautiful, or even called ugly, are routinely abused and ostracized. Social prejudice based on appearance is not new – we have seen in earlier chapters the lazy shorthand about ugly people being immoral or sinful. But appearance-related bullying has increased in the past twenty years – and that is directly related to social media, and the perceived availability of cosmetic surgery.

The British actor Adam Pearson lives with neurofibromatosis, a condition that causes benign vascular tumours to appear and multiply all over the face. When I interviewed him about his role in the film *A Different Man* (2024), he said people routinely ask why he doesn't have surgery to remove his tumours. His response was simple – 'Bruh, this is after surgery.' Adam's life involves – has always involved – regular and frequent visits to the surgeon he has had since childhood. His tumours cannot be removed. Neurofibromatosis tumours do not exist just on the skin, at surface level. They develop in the brain, the spinal cord and the nerves.

And anyway, why should Adam have surgery purely to meet other people's aesthetic expectations?

One of the reasons why we don't have face transplants in the U.K. is, as we will see in chapter nine, because the idea that surgery offers a quick fix puts pressure on everyone to go under the knife. Dallas Wiens, a face-transplant recipient from Texas, told me that, when he lost his own face in an electrical accident, strangers would yell: 'Who the hell does that guy think he is?' and 'How dare he leave the house without a mask?'

The American Society of Plastic Surgeons has found that childhood bullying, which might start in the playground but now accompanies young people everywhere on their smartphones, encourages thoughts of cosmetic surgery from adolescence. And we can understand why; young people with 'visible difference' – or, to use the legal and surgical term, 'disfigurement' – are three times more likely to be bullied than other children, and three times more likely to have their image circulated without consent.

And yet, rather than being invited to speak to other patients who have gone under the knife, or asked what they are *really* hoping to change, prospective patients are simply encouraged to do their own research; to find the best surgeon, much as they would a good builder. The Royal College of Surgeons of England is a professional rather than a statutory regulatory body. It sets standards and offers certification in cosmetic surgery but has no powers over many non-surgical interventions.

The Royal College of Surgeons was established in 1800, since when much has changed but a lot has stayed the same. There were no female surgeons in 1800, and plastic surgery remains a male-dominated profession, though that is starting to change. Only around 20 per cent of plastic surgeons in the U.K. are female (15 per cent in the U.S.); by contrast over 90 per cent of plastic-surgery patients are female, in the U.S. and the U.K. alike.

Such statistics show the power imbalances in the patient–practitioner relationship. It is mostly men who are 'improving' women, whether those women are cis or trans or non-binary; patriarchal beliefs about appearance do not just reinforce beauty standards – they shape them. And isn't that reminiscent of how differently male and female faces have always been treated in art, photography and popular culture?

Conventional gender-affirmation surgeries include the reshaping of the forehead, brows, nose, cheeks and jaw; the reduction of an Adam's apple; the moving of hairlines to create smaller foreheads; and enlargement to the lips and cheekbones in the pursuit of a more stereotypically feminine appearance. For female to male transitions, testosterone makes the skin oilier and thicker, jawlines can be made larger and more pronounced, brows heavier.

Meanwhile, Botox and fillers are so normalized that they are referred to as 'lunchtime tweakments', and many cosmetic interventions – including fillers and Botox in the U.K. – can be given by people without qualifications. This, even though they still carry considerable risk – badly administered injectables can lead to blindness, scarring and paralysis. In an independent review in 2013, the NHS Medical Director Bruce Keogh said that people had 'no more protection or redress' when having injectables that could make them blind, or facially paralyse them, 'than [when] buying a ballpoint pen or a toothbrush'.

Some clinics that use manipulated images on social media might also inflate reviews on sites such as Trustpilot to make sure they get 5-star ratings. Potential patients need to dig deeper to find the truth, and there are complex reasons why that might not happen – including both the patient–practitioner power imbalance and confirmation bias. By the time a person sees a surgeon, they may be so desperate for surgery, and so overwhelmed by choices, that they do not share what they are really feeling. The desire for cosmetic surgery, at least in Europe, carries layers of guilt and shame.

On the one hand people – women – are encouraged to look their best and shamed for not doing so; on the other, it is seen as self-indulgent vanity to go under the knife just to look good. This, then, presents a series of double binds for patient-consumers: by treating the face as a commodity to be improved, people are expected to be realistic – but not honest with their surgeons; to look good – but not be vain; to appear younger than their age – but never 'mutton dressed as lamb'.

And what of the racial politics? A Eurocentric ideal that is unattainable for most is akin to cultural genocide: noses are trimmed and narrowed and turned up, chins are shortened, eyes widened and skin lightened, as though genetic diversity were a pathology. Nothing, it seems, can disturb the quest for the perfect Hollywood face.

We must ask – where is this limited model of beauty coming from? The obvious answer is from history, from the inherited physiognomic and Victorian biases discussed in this book.

There is also an 'anchor bias' in modern science, which means it's difficult to dislodge the first thing that we learn about a topic. In modern evolutionary psychology, traces of outdated bias about race still appear in links to Darwinian theory though the very idea of race as a category has been debunked. It is not just anchor bias at work, but also deeply held and implicit beliefs about the world.

Western economic and social systems are committed to the

idea of the survival of the fittest, which justifies wealth and power being consolidated in the hands of a small number of largely white, largely male individuals. As with patriarchy, it is convenient if that practice is seen as 'natural', justified by science and even religion, as we see in the rhetoric of the American Republican Party. Rhetoric matters more than accuracy.

Let me give you an example of how sexist and racist ideas get diluted and reproduced under the name of science. In 2023 I interviewed a leading computer scientist about facial appearance; I was researching how appearance ideals established by the classical and Victorian periods are normalized and reproduced. Not to worry, the computer scientist told me; today, it is possible to determine an absolute standard by which beauty is calculated. He explained that there was a simple, mathematical formula, which came from the ancient Greeks.

I held my breath as the computer scientist explained how he and a colleague had used the golden ratio to create a computer software program that could easily assess who was beautiful and who was not. There was no bias, he said, since the program could generate a series of algorithms that were based on objective mathematical proportions.

I asked the computer scientist how those algorithms were determined, and he frowned. 'We put in information.' Yes, but what information? He looked confused, as though the answer should be obvious: 'The usual. You know, women that are generally accepted as beautiful. Like, *FHM* and *GQ* readers' polls.'

I sighed – at the error, and the obliviousness. The information being used to assess an objective measure for beauty by scientists who should know better was based on established European viewpoints. We see the same kind of bias in facial-recognition systems and even foetal scanning, as we will see. When computer algorithms are trained with selective rather than diverse data, they inherit those biases and reinforce prejudiced ideas as fact.

The computer scientist hadn't noticed that they were excluding people of colour, people with disabilities, people with unusual or different faces. And perhaps he didn't notice because this practice is routinely carried out.

'Greek mathematics reveal most beautiful woman on the planet', announced the *Daily Mail* in 2019. That woman was Bella Hadid, who despite being Muslim and mixed race – her mother is Dutch, her father Palestinian – conforms to European beauty standards. This is largely because she had a nose job at the age of fourteen, which she later regretted, telling *Vogue* magazine, 'I wish I had kept the nose of my ancestors.'

It is a safe bet that with that ancestral nose, no matter how beautiful, Hadid would not have been on the cover of so many Western magazines.

In 2024 the *Daily Mail* announced a new forerunner in 'the science of beauty': the actor Anya Taylor-Joy, who was the world's most attractive woman 'according to Golden Ratio of Beauty Phi'. This time, Hadid came second, followed by the actor Margot Robbie.

Where do tabloids like the *Daily Mail* get their data? From the research of 'British scientists', they say – a source that turns out to be a famous doctor –, a cosmetic surgeon with a Harley Street practice. Much that is published online today appears under the banner of 'research', a term that once implied systematic and rigorous inquiry but is now often used loosely to lend authority to selective or commercially driven claims.

The golden ratio has been revived several times since the classical period. Not only did Leonardo da Vinci incorporate elements of Euclid's theory into the *Mona Lisa* and the *Vitruvian Man*, but also its thread of order and proportion was implicit in the development of race theory in the eighteenth century. Then the German anthropologist and white supremacist Christoph Meiners argued, in *The Outline of History of Mankind*, that only white people could be beautiful; their faces were better proportioned, their bodies were softer and more sensitive.

For the Victorians, the golden ratio was less important than other forms of measurement. They cared about hierarchies, health and fitness, in ways that could be attached to Darwinian thought and evolutionary biology. Beauty standards became tied to ideas of racial superiority and evolution rather more than to ancient mathematical or aesthetic ideals. And while white faces were seen as beautiful, Black faces showed primitivism (linked to Neanderthals), threat (akin to criminals) and ridicule; the latter was most evident when white people 'blacked up' for comedic effect.

Blackface proliferated after the end of the international slave trade. The ubiquity of big-lipped, frizzy-wigged minstrel shows, cartoons and circuses made a mockery of the faces, emotions and experiences of Black people, and made Blackness a source of caricature rather than humanity. Jewish people have similarly been stereotyped and caricatured over the centuries as hook-nosed and greedy, as we saw in our discussion of photography. This is not accidental: by depicting some people's faces as less human, particular groups are denied common empathy. It becomes easier, through that lens, for individuals and groups to be denied human rights, and human understanding.

In the later twentieth century, the idea of the body beautiful still drew on the physical ideals celebrated by the Nazis. This included an interest in the 'master race', in order and symmetry and in the eugenic principles pioneered by Francis Galton, whom we met in an earlier chapter. The Nazis did not explicitly use the golden ratio when they catalogued the perfect Aryan face, but Hitler was so enamoured of the Greek statue known as *Discobolus* – the 'discus-thrower' – for its order, proportion and beauty that he purchased it in 1938.

The golden ratio has had something of a rebirth in the early twenty-first century, alongside the upward swing of cosmetic surgery and platforms like Instagram and TikTok, feeding off each other in the quest for and display of the perfect face. We know that cosmetic procedures increased after the pandemic of 2019, with all that screen culture, but even before the pandemic, the number of cosmetic surgeries was rising. The American Society of Plastic Surgeons records 12.5 million cosmetic procedures of all kinds in the U.S. in 2009, but as many as 27 million by 2023.

Much of that increase can be attributed to cosmetic surgeons using digital platforms to sell their services; according to one research study, nearly 20 per cent of one million posts analysed were created by cosmetic surgeons.

This brings us back to the @estemedistanbultr affair. We have seen why people might desire the quick fix of cosmetic treatments, for they offer so much promise. Cosmetic surgeons regularly use the golden ratio in promoting their services: it offers an easy, apparently objective measurement system for deciding exactly what is 'wrong' with your face. It's not just my judgement, the cosmetic surgeon can say, this is a standard that has been used for thousands of years. The murky history of facial measurements is hidden beneath the guise of classical wisdom and given the label of objectivity.

It reminds me of an unpleasant encounter I had in 2022 with a small group of male European cosmetic researchers who said that they, too, knew the formula for female beauty. They were developing an AI tool to model 'ideal' facial proportions for potential patients, and we met online to discuss a possible collaboration with my Interface project at King's College London, where I study the history and meanings of the human face.

Mindful of my earlier exchange with the computer scientist, I asked for more information about how the group's formula for beauty was calculated. They told me that they input the data. Then I pressed further and asked, 'What data?' explaining that I was interested in how cultural bias shapes computer algorithms. This did not go down well; the lead researcher told me that his team knew precisely what beauty was – that some of them had PhDs, and others were trained as artists, and anyway, the information I asked for was protected as intellectual property.

I was conscious that I had crossed an invisible line threatening their white-coated authority, and that the leader of the team didn't like it. His expression hardened. 'If you were a patient of mine, for instance, I might tell you that you are sixty per cent beautiful,' he said. 'Perhaps you would like me to tell you what is wrong with your face?'

I did not. Nor did I tell him what I thought was wrong with *his* face, largely because I forgot it the moment that I switched off the computer. Sometimes prosopagnosia has its uses.

I am not alone in finding this presumption of male surgical authority, and the emphasis on the golden ratio, problematic. One American surgeon, Stephen R. Marquardt, set himself up as a leading authority on beauty and facial analysis, and created a 3D mask based on its principles in order to make life easier to determine what needs 'correcting'. The so-called 'Marquardt Beauty Mask' is based on classical models, and allegedly universal, but unsuitable for non-European populations. Korean surgeons, for instance, rejected the mask as unusable for their client base; Thai surgeons also found it didn't measure up – even when used on the face of Miss Universe Thailand; South Indian researchers drew the same conclusions. The mask might be easy for surgeons to use, but that does not make it a single universal standard for beauty.

And yet the visual language of the golden ratio seems almost to have been designed for social media: TikTok has a 'face filter' so people can judge their own faces, and there are nearly 20,000 videos with the hashtag 'Golden Ratio'. On Instagram it's the same – there are more than 600,000 posts #goldenratio, most of which include people discussing the 'ideal face'.

Other troubling face myths and ideals are pedalled by digital platforms, as part of the global homogenization of beauty standards, including filters that lighten the skin and Westernize faces. Actual physical skin bleaching has long been an issue in Africa, Latin America, India and the Middle East, directly related to the history of facial prejudice we've explored throughout this book. In India alone, skin-whitening creams account for 40–50 per cent of the cosmetics market. Cosmetic surgery around the world also relates to the Western ideal; in Venezuela, there is demand for thinner, 'European' noses; and in Korea, for double-eyelid surgery, a procedure that creates an upper-eyelid crease.

We are witnessing the global standardization of faces according to one cultural ideal. The same forces that drove colonial expansion – the belief that European ways of looking and being were superior – now operate through Instagram filters and surgery clinics. It's cultural imperialism with a scalpel.

As with disability activism and Black beauty standards, not every woman is looking to conform to conventional facial aesthetics. The French multimedia and performance artist ORLAN, for example, underwent multiple cosmetic surgeries in the 1990s to critique ideals of female beauty. ORLAN made an artwork out of her own face: she modelled her forehead on Leonardo's *Mona Lisa*, her chin on Botticelli's *Venus*, her eyes on François Pascal Simon Gérard's *Psyche* and her mouth on Gustave Moreau's *Europa*. Each element of beauty was chosen because of the stories we associate with them, rather than because of the parts themselves.

ORLAN stayed awake for all these operations, and the designers Paco Rabanne and Issey Miyake gave her clothes to wear on the operating table. Around her, people read poetry and played music. ORLAN was both observer and observed, canvas and artist, for an art series that was filmed and broadcast around the world: 'The Reincarnation of Sainte-ORLAN'.

Most of us do not curate our faces as controversially and provocatively as ORLAN. I have focused in this chapter on the pursuit of the perfect face, but many older people aren't looking for a radical transformation – they want to recapture their youth, feeling the weight of that loss, perhaps after a lifetime of kids, bills, work and stress. Cosmetic enhancement in this context is framed by surgeons, and by individuals themselves, not as the pursuit of an Instagram ideal, but as a form of self-care, especially for mothers after their children have left home.

This is a different kind of surrendering not just to consumer culture but also to the belief – or desire to believe – that if we change our face, we can change our life. Nowhere is youth celebrated more than in the Global North, as a shorthand for individualism, freedom and beauty. The desire for youth, as for beauty, is seen as natural, rather than as a reflection of how culturally invisible older people, especially women, can become.

Perhaps cosmetic surgery is inevitable today, now we have the skills, the materials and the desire. And there is no judgement here: I know plenty of brilliant feminists of all shapes, sizes, genders and colours who have gone under the knife. I also know a smaller number of caring, ethical and principled cosmetic surgeons.

But apart from anything else, I wonder whether our focus on the visuals – and on the need to look a certain way – has done a disservice to the many things that make a person beautiful – the way they move, their scent, the crinkled eyes that show they laugh easily, a fleeting openness that can't be captured by a measurement or static image. It is often natural, imperfect beauty, of the kind destroyed by homogeneity, that makes a person irresistible – a wonky nose, for instance, or an idiosyncratic hairline.

As a teenager, I was almost exclusively attracted to men with interesting teeth: the tennis ace Ivan Lendl, David Bowie, Freddie Mercury; a boy called Stuart who rode a moped. I was gutted when Bowie perfected his teeth in later life. I wasn't interested in jocks or film stars, and I wouldn't have contemplated surgery to look like Debbie Harry or Kim Wilde. I would have liked to look like them, sure, but I had no frame of reference, in the 1980s, that it was possible. Nor did I have to endure the constant promotion of images of gorgeous celebrities, except when I chose to go to the corner shop and flick through glossy magazines. A friend suggested that perhaps this was because I grew up in rural Wales and not West London, where omnipresent billboards and advertising would have some young people thinking: if only.

There is, however, something different at work today, when social media is the principal means of communication for teenagers, as well as for entertainment, lifestyle and health. There is a proven relationship between the low self-esteem found in young people who use Instagram and the desire for cosmetic surgery. That's why the Australian Society of Aesthetic Plastic Surgeons supported regulations by their government from 2023, putting limits on what cosmetic surgeons can advertise online. Any suggestion that surgery is 'quick' or 'simple' or 'gentle' has been banned, and surgeons cannot promise a psychological fix through a physical change – so no more talk about restoring a 'youthful' complexion or making people 'happier and healthier'.

Cosmetic surgery does not, on balance, make people happier – even if the results are objectively good. As much as we think a procedure might change our life, we are likely to be disappointed. As the psychologist Nichola Rumsey, the founder of the Centre for Appearance Research, told me, it might 'give you a slight lift, metaphorically and literally, but the effects are temporary and will probably leave you wanting more'. And surgery can be addictive; a nip here can lead to a tuck there; before we know it, we are in the 'uncanny valley'. This term was coined by the Japanese roboticist, Masahiro Mori, to explain the unease experienced when we encounter characters that are almost, but not quite, human.

The uncanny valley brings contempt and derision, even revulsion. The same tabloids that celebrate homogenized beauties swiftly condemn those who go too far. Jocelyn Périsset, the Swiss socialite billionaire, was famed for her feline-influenced cosmetic enhancements. Media outlets called her 'cat woman', and 'the Bride of Wildenstein'. Her surgery love affair started when she and her husband, Alec Wildenstein, had eyelifts to look more refreshed. Once she got the bug, she couldn't stop, according to *Vanity Fair*: 'She was crazy,' Alec said, 'she was thinking she could fix her face like a piece of furniture. Skin does not work that way. But she wouldn't listen.'

A more recent example is the British model and reality star Katie Price, who has spoken openly about her love of consumerism and cosmetic surgery. As well as several breast lifts and liposuction, she is said to have had multiple facial treatments: Botox, fillers, laser resurfacing, ear pinning, lip and eye lifts, chemical peels and a facelift. Strangers take to their keyboards to tell her she has 'gone too far', that she is a whore, a bad mother, crazy, a drug addict, and so on. But what is her crime? She views her face (and her body) as commodities to change and adapt as her mood dictates. And isn't that the promise of consumerism – that it is a choice?

We will always be judged, it seems, no matter what we do with our faces, and what we do with our faces is complex. They are malleable and moveable; making the face *immoveable* might be the point of Botox – but at what cost? It is how we move our faces, in smiling, kissing, talking, singing, seeing, smelling, touching, feeling, eating, drinking, connecting to others – that is more important than what we look like, isn't it?

Our connection to the faces of others starts from birth – perhaps even earlier, as the next chapter shows. When we search out the faces of foetuses, we are increasingly influenced by the same desire for perfection found on Instagram. We are also influenced by the desire to know, to capture, to image and to classify faces in ways that echo our Victorian ancestors. Nowhere is safe from the camera lens, it turns out, not even the womb.

5.
Grown

Legend has it that Bartholomew the Apostle, also known as Nathanael, once cried out *in utero*. That's not the only mysterious mythology around birth; Alexander the Great's mother, Olympias, claimed that in her dream Zeus appeared in the form of a serpent, impregnating her, making Alexander the son of a god. Jesus Christ was conceived through immaculate conception, Mary made pregnant by the Holy Spirit. And John the Baptist leapt at the sound of Mary's voice while he was still in the womb.

As with other mystical happenings, such stories can't be proven, except that there have been cases of foetuses crying in the womb like Bartholomew. Vagitus uterinus is a rare but documented event in which a foetus breathes air because an amniotic sac has been torn. It is far more common for foetuses to cry silently within sealed sacs, their faces moving to practise the expressions they will need in the world of the human.

Historically it makes sense that such myths surrounded pregnancy and birth, partly to evidence the predestined specialness of apostles, leaders and gods, but also because birth was such a mysterious process. Who knew *how* a baby developed in the womb, since one couldn't see it happen?

And babies' faces, once they were born, didn't receive any special artistic attention, at least until the Renaissance; in medieval portraiture they were merely figurative and looked like adults. Physiognomists were not even interested in young faces until adulthood, when every part of the face had meaning – even the philtrum, that small groove at the centre of our top lip.

It was the ancient Greeks who gave the philtrum its name; the word means 'love charm', because it was thought to entice lovers. In the eighteenth century, the Swiss physiognomist Johann Kaspar Lavater claimed an overly long philtrum showed 'want of prudence'. Its shape and length could, for other writers, signify chastity, sexuality and even stupidity.

We might not judge people by their philtrum today – at least consciously; most of us don't know its name, let alone why it exists. But stories survive; in John Huston's 1948 film *Key Largo*, Frank 'Soldier' McCloud, played by Humphrey Bogart, says that a newborn comes into the world with all the wisdom of heaven and earth. But an angel presses the child's lips together with their finger; from that moment they cannot share their knowledge with anyone. This story is a variation on a Jewish legend from the Babylonian Talmud; there, an angel teaches the Torah to every foetus *in utero*, before smacking it on the mouth.

That an infant was born all-knowing, but forgetting, has been a popular idea for centuries (and it survives – how often young babies are called 'old souls' today because their faces seem solemn and wise!). Exactly which parts of our inner selves are learned, and which we were born with, has been debated since the philosopher John Locke declared our minds a 'tabula rasa' or blank slate. We are less uncertain about our faces, which are shaped in the womb by our environment, and the cells of our ancestors.

And our faces grew, for centuries, unseen. Men might have governed but women knew the secrets of the womb and the paternity of their foetuses. The medical concept of 'maternal influence' dictated that it was the emotions, thoughts and behaviour of a mother that influenced a newborn's appearance. What she ate and drank, desired or ruminated over, mattered. One sniff of a strawberry could result in a birthmark on a child's cheek, and many cases of infant disability were blamed on the imprudence of expectant mothers.

In 1726, Mary Toft, a poor woman from Surrey, claimed maternal influence to trick doctors into believing she had given birth to a litter of rabbits. Mary said she was working in the fields when she was distracted by a rabbit. She and her fellow labourers tried to catch it for their supper, but they failed, and Mary miscarried. Her disappointed longing for that rabbit was supposed to have led to a subsequent birth of twelve dead rabbits; Mary's testimony was supported by her doctor, who had pulled the animal parts from her body himself.

This extraordinary story reached the ears of the king and court and involved some of the country's most eminent surgeons in a debate; could this monstrous tale be true? Eventually, the hoax was revealed – Mary confessed that with the help of a friend she had stuffed her vagina with parts of dead rabbits to make money from the affair, this being the age of freak shows. Instead, she was imprisoned for being a 'cheat and imposter', and her publicly humiliated surgeon was fined.

Mary's tale reached the courts because of male anxiety about female rebellion at a time when midwifery was becoming a male profession. There had long been patriarchal distrust about the birth process – including the appearance of monstrous and misshapen offspring.

How could a mere woman be entrusted to gestate a child? And how could a man ever be certain that a beloved son and heir was not another man's, or even a changeling, left by a supernatural being? It was the 1800s before the idea of 'phenotypes' developed (that is, recognizable similarities in nose or ear shape). Before then, there was less discussion of family resemblances.

Today a doubting father might demand a DNA test if he were not satisfied by the passing on of 'jug ears' or a family nose. But scientific paternity analysis wasn't possible before blood-type analysis in the 1920s.

Early modern scientists did not have access to such modern testing, but as early as the 1700s there was dissatisfaction at the invisibility of the womb. Enlightenment science wanted to see things to believe them – vision was the most important sense; it was associated with men and with reason.

Women, whose work sat at the intersection of life and death – as birthers, healers, midwives, carers for the sick and the dying – could easily find themselves accused of treachery or witchcraft when things went wrong. Women represented the non-visual senses, and the natural world that needed to be tamed.

The rise of male midwifery, which gradually pushed women out of their traditional roles, was an assertion of patriarchal power. Some male midwives and surgeons had attended European births since the 1600s, but in the eighteenth century, male midwives and anatomists opened and displayed women's bodies in ways that were previously unthinkable.

The use of obstetric forceps was central to this transformation – not merely because they were medically superior to other invasive procedures, but because they gave male practitioners a technological advantage that traditional female midwives could not match. Forceps became both a genuine medical tool and a powerful symbol of male scientific authority over women's bodies and the birth process.

William Hunter, Physician Extraordinary to Queen Charlotte, wife of George III, published *The Anatomy of the Gravid Uterus* in 1774; while his brother John was the most eminent pathologist in Britain, William set out to remove obstetrics from the midwives and establish it as a distinct medical specialism. He did this by offering graphic anatomical images of inside the womb; this enabled comparisons to be made between dead specimens, and offered insights that traditional midwives, guided only by what they could see on the outside (and by touch, smell and hearing), could not.

Readers might remember from chapter one how difficult it was to obtain bodies for dissection in the eighteenth century; this was the world of Burke and Hare, the infamous body snatchers of early nineteenth-century Edinburgh. It has been alleged that Hunter knowingly bought the bodies of murdered poor women, since how else did he end up with so many pregnant women to dissect? We will probably never know the truth.

What is important here is what Hunter did with those bodies – or rather, with what was inside them. Unlike later images of the pregnant womb, we do not see the face of the foetus; Hunter's exceptionally detailed plates – made by the Dutch artist Jan van Rymsdyk – focused on the anatomy of the woman's body. This gave rise to painstaking reproductions of the muscles and veins of the womb, which was stripped of its outer layers; when we see the foetus, it is not personalized; its body is turned away from the viewer, with its face squished against the womb lining or pressed inside the birth canal.

These are violent images of pregnancy by today's terms – the expectant mother's legs are amputated at the thigh, her genitals and innards exposed as though she is an invisible container for the baby-making machine within.

Did Hunter's work enhance medical knowledge of pregnancy? Yes. Did that knowledge save lives? Almost certainly. But it also diminished women's autonomy over their own bodies, and over the birth process, in ways that were characteristic of the time.

It is a myth that Louis XIV was solely responsible for women lying on their backs to give birth, thus ensuring no baby-swaps took place, but reputedly he did enjoy the spectacle. The prone position made it easier for man-midwives and surgeons to view the birth and use forceps – a relatively new piece of kit with a technological edge that reassured wealthy patients. So, birth became a more public event, and the womb became more accessible, but the foetus and its face were not yet centre stage.

Why so little interest in the foetus? Technically, it has no legal rights or personhood until it is born – at least in the U.K.; in other countries, including the U.S., things are less clear because of jurisdictional differences; extending legal rights to foetuses or embryos is an ongoing debate.

I believe that personhood, emotionally, if not legally, is expected to have a face. Not a generic, mini-adult face, as we saw in medieval plates of Jesus *in utero*, but a realistic, identifiable, infant face – of the kind used in modern anti-abortion campaigns.

And we can have that now, thanks to medical technology. Foetal imaging has exposed many secrets of the womb, showing for instance how the face fits together – and where the philtrum comes in (fig. 20).

First, the two facial nerves develop in the third week, one on each side of the head, and they send signals between the brain and the face and allow facial expressions, talking, tasting and tear production. In its early stages, the human face looks like any other mammal, bird, or amphibian embryo, all of which evolved from fish; with eyes on the sides of

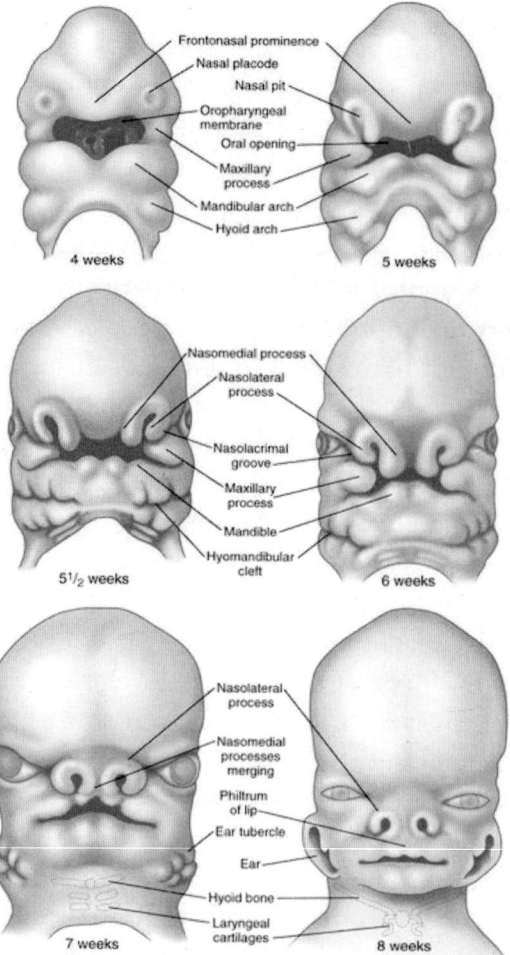

20. Unknown artist, *The Puzzle of the Face*, 2024.

the head, which gradually move to the centre. The top lip and the jaw begin like gills, on the sides of the neck, while the nostrils descend from the top. As the face forms, so does the philtrum or 'medial cleft', a far less romantic name than 'love charm', which is common in mammals that give birth to live young; it marks the point at which the sides of the face join, like a puzzle, between weeks five and eight of gestation.

If the puzzle of the face doesn't fit together during this critical stage of development, then it never will. That's what happened to

Yahya El Jabaly, whom the media chose to call the 'boy without a face'. Yahya was born in 2012 in a village near Tangiers. For an unknown reason, his face did not fit together at the critical stage: he was born with a hole in his face where his nose should have been, no eyes, and an upper jaw that turned upwards and outwards. As a result, Yahya was unable to speak, and since the upper part of his skull had not formed, part of his brain was only covered by skin. After a Facebook appeal for help, he underwent years of reconstructive surgery in Melbourne; many people, especially in the Global South, do not have access to the kinds of facial reconstruction surgery that we take for granted in the Global North.

Facial disfigurement, or visible difference, to use the term preferred by disability advocates, affects 10 per cent of the world's population. Many of these are congenital facial problems, such as cleft lip, once known as 'hare lip'. This term was not descriptive, it was a reference to maternal influence. Mothers of babies with cleft lips were popularly believed to have stumbled across a hare when pregnant – less dramatic versions of the Mary Toft affair. Today, about one in 700 babies worldwide is born with a cleft palate, with higher rates where prenatal care and nutrition are limited.

Bullying is commonplace for people with 'different' faces, as we saw in the previous chapter. In the past, this was justified by scripture and science. The Book of Leviticus, first published in 300 BCE, warned that 'one who has a mutilated face' wasn't welcome in holy places; this applied to other forms of physical disability, for as we have seen, the body reflected the state of the soul. The nineteenth-century revival of physiognomy reinforced the link; Lavater, the physiognomist who was preoccupied with philtrum length, claimed that 'the morally worst [were the] the most deformed'.

Even today, when we know anyone can be injured, and that faces can grow in different ways, we lack compassion. Thrillers, horror movies and even children's literature rely on disfigurement as a shorthand for evil: James Bond's *Skyfall* (Raoul Silva), *No Time to Die* (Lyutsifer Safin) and *Casino Royale* (Le Chiffre); Darth Vader in *Star*

Wars; Freddy Krueger in *A Nightmare on Elm Street*; Voldemort in *Harry Potter*. Social stigma is often the worst part of visible difference.

During the pandemic, many people with visible difference talked to me about the relief of wearing a mask; for the first time, they could walk down the street without stares and chat to strangers without them flinching or looking away. While most people sighed with relief when mask regulations were lifted, those with visible difference were once again socially shunned.

Visible difference in the womb is harder to detect. Most prenatal ultrasound can't tell when the face is growing differently. Ultrasound is quite an old technology, developed during the Second World War from techniques of navigation through sound. Strangely it wasn't used in medicine before the 1960s, when its job was to measure the diameter of a foetus's head. The pioneer of that use was Ian Donald, an obstetrician from Glasgow, the city where William Hunter studied.

Alongside ultrasound came photography. The Edwardians built on the Victorian way of knowing and classifying the world, and the first films of a living foetus were made between 1932 and 1963 – by Davenport Hooker, an anatomist from the University of Pittsburgh. Since there was no way of accessing the interior of women's wombs at that time, Hooker made an agreement with a local hospital to film aborted foetuses while they were still alive. He planned to plot embryonic development in the same way that other scientists had plotted human evolution.

Hooker filmed 149 foetuses, ranging in age from six to forty-five weeks. He was interested in when movement and sensation happened and found that by eleven and a half weeks the face was sensitive to touch. By fourteen and a half weeks it could open and close its mouth, scowl and swallow.

Some of Hooker's images, including that of a five-month-old foetus published in *Look* magazine in 1962, contributed to new visual and biomedical ideas of foetuses as baby-like and autonomous human entities. And it anticipated the work of the Swedish photographer Lennart Nilsson, who finally made the foetal face public.

In the 1950s, Nilsson already had a national reputation for his environmentalism and photojournalism, with essays such as 'A Midwife in Lapland' (1945) and 'Polar Bear Hunting in Spitzbergen' (1947). For years he harboured an ambition to record the physical development of the foetus in the womb, but it seemed a technological impossibility – how to get inside the womb without hurting the foetus? And how to get images of a sufficiently high resolution to track foetal growth?

In the pursuit of answers, Nilsson hired the German company Karl Storz and the Swedish company Jungners Optiska in Stockholm, which manufactured macro-lenses and wide-angled optics. He began to experiment with extreme close-ups using endoscopes – long, thin tubes with lights and cameras attached. His results were published in 1965 as a photographic essay for *Life* magazine. 'Drama of Life before Birth' charted the stages of human reproduction, from fertilization to birth, for the first time and in glorious technicolour.

Unsurprisingly, the images made Nilsson famous. They also marked an important cultural moment in the history of the face, and of humanity itself. For at that time, people were simultaneously reaching for the stars – the Russians launched Sputnik 1 in 1957 and the U.S. and Soviet Union soon after engaged in the Space Race – and reaching into the most intimate spaces of the human body.

Nilsson's images echoed this duality, using the cultural motifs of space exploration in his pictures of the foetus. When the *Life* issue hit the news stands in 1965, just four years before the first U.S. moon landing, Russian and American astronauts had already walked in space, and millions of dollars were being invested in American college programmes.

Nilsson's tiny foetal astronaut floated in a sea of amniotic fluid, against a backdrop of stars (fig. 21): the frontiers of birth, like those of space, seemed to have been conquered at last. At just eighteen weeks the foetus seemed to be sleeping peacefully, its small button nose in profile, its tiny hands clasped in front of its chest. To the right of the image, the umbilical cord is attached to the amniotic sac via the placenta, just as those brave astronauts were tethered to their spacecraft. Nilsson's images helped *Life* sell out its eight million copies in just four days.

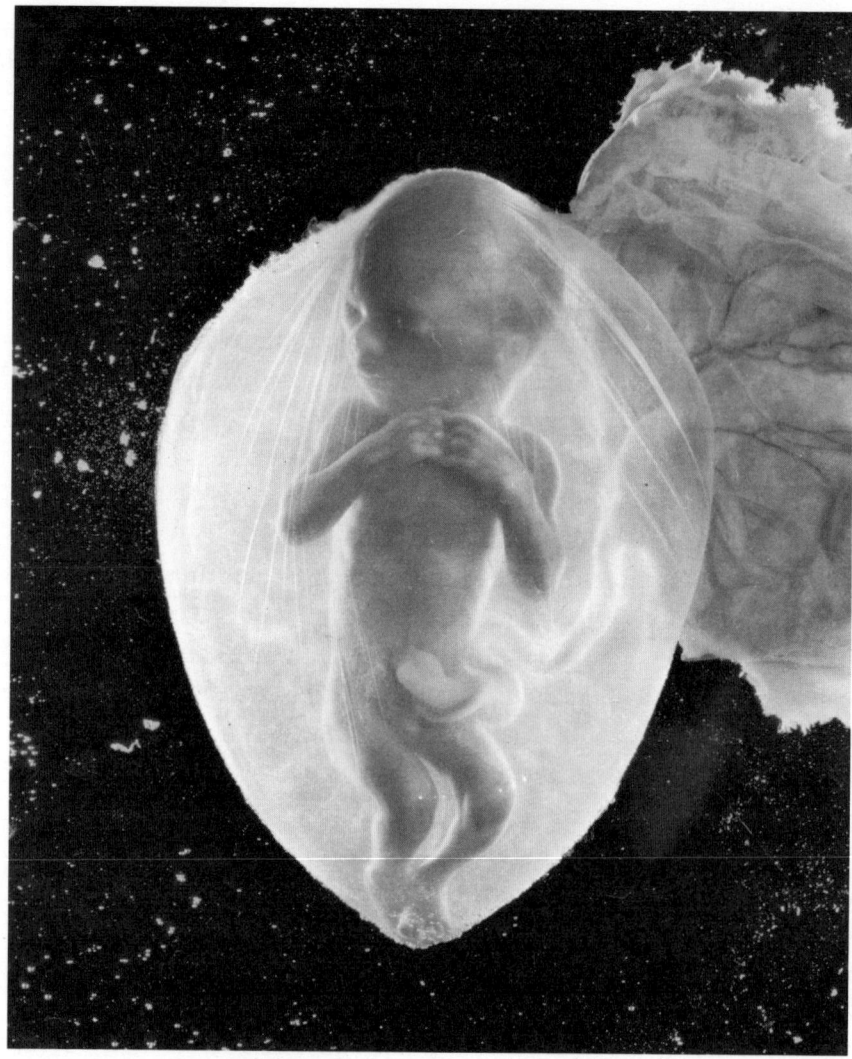

21. Lennart Nilsson, on the cover of *Life* magazine, 1965.

Nilsson's images were as path-breaking as Hunter's images had been, but markedly different in aim and approach. Hunter's were designed for medical professionals, Nilsson's for the public. Hunter had no interest in depicting the foetal face, but Nilsson recognized its emotive power.

In an interview with PBS news, Nilsson explained how it had

taken him twelve years to get the story. The first images he had taken with the endoscope were of legs, hands, feet and sex organs, parts of the foetus that showed its development but not the most important part. What he really wanted to capture was the face.

Also, unlike Hunter, whose plates were arranged in reverse chronological order (from a woman who died at nine months' gestation to one who died at five weeks), Nilsson's images were placed chronologically, from fertilization to birth. The sequence of images and imagery, the descriptions of the foetus and the focus on the foetus as an individual make it clear that it was the star of the show. It also had a story: by three months it was a 5.6 cm-long girl, 'with noticeably human traits'; at four months, she had a well-developed face and was showing 'individual characteristics'.

The telling of the foetus's growth gave her a sense of individual identity and momentum, without any reference to the woman's body that was vital for its development. The story takes readers from the 'miracle' of conception to the enthusiastic arms of the baby's parents, as featured in the book that followed the photo essay: *A Child is Born*. That book was published in forty countries and was thought to be so culturally significant that it was sent into space in 1977 with NASA's Voyager time-capsule probes.

For the first time a foetus was being visually presented not as a medical specimen or an anatomical curiosity but as the protagonist in its own story, and with features that encouraged the emotional engagement of readers. This marks an obvious cultural shift since the time of William Hunter; had the physician wanted to show the face of the foetus then he would have done – van Rymsdyk was more than expert at capturing realism and working within difficult physical parameters.

But it was Nilsson who chose to capture the delicate strands of fine hair, lanugo, that covered the foetus's cheeks and lashes, the marbled blue veins beneath the surface of its eyelids, the miniature thumb caught between pale lips. He sought out the baby in these images, depicting what the foetus could become, rather than simply what it was. He documented the journey of the parents, too, in *A Child is Born*; like every image of a foetus photographed by Nilsson, those parents were white. This was in keeping with the racially homogeneous nature of Sweden in the 1960s, in which more than 99 per cent of the population was Caucasian, but also with the ingrained traditions of Western medicine.

Despite being innovative in technological use, Nilsson's photo essay was therefore traditional in scope. It implicitly celebrated the nuclear family and was published at a time when women's rights were under dispute. There were few legal abortions in Sweden in the 1960s; they had been permitted for social and medical grounds from the 1940s, but they were not yet available on demand.

Nilsson's images were also used by opponents of abortion, not only in Sweden but internationally, though he claimed to be ignorant of the fact. And you can see why the images were influential. Not only did they give personhood to the foetus by focusing on its human face and individual quest – echoing humankind's parallel

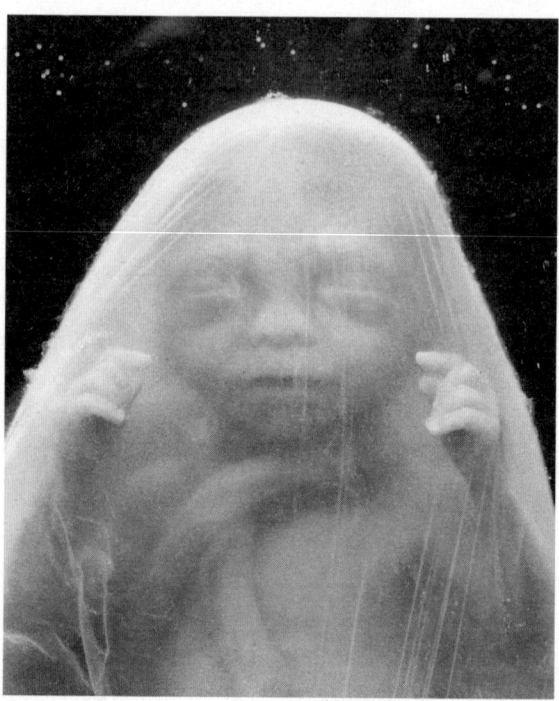

22. Lennart Nilsson, *Foetus at eighteen weeks*, 1965.

quest in space – they also resonated with spiritual imagery. Intentionally or not, the eighteen-week foetus, with its embryonic sac transparently visible (fig. 22), is reminiscent of the Veiled Virgin, a nineteenth-century bust by the Italian sculptor Giovanni Strazza (fig. 23). The viewer did not need to know that artwork to grasp the association; the veil has a long cultural association in Western art with innocence and virtue.

If we look more closely at Nilsson's image, however, we see the umbilical cord wrapped around the foetus's neck; it is not a veil but a shroud. Because that foetus, like all but one of Nilsson's subjects, was dead; just as Hunter's had been.

Here lies one of the most profound ironies in the history of foetal imaging. Photographing a living foetus *in utero* is extremely risky: pushing anything, including an endoscope, into the womb carries a risk of infection and miscarriage. Nilsson took just one image of

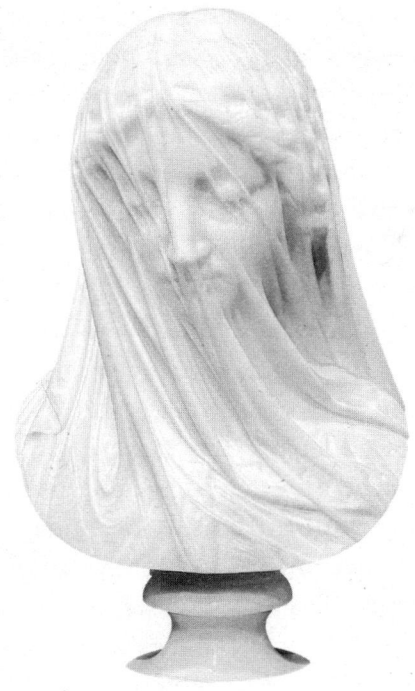

23. Giovanni Strazza, *The Veiled Virgin*, early 1850s.

a foetus *in utero*: 'very sharp, of just the face, the head of the fetus inside the womb'.

But he had seen dead embryos in jars in a medical office; they were kept there so that doctors could show them to pregnant women, to deter them from having abortions. Inspired by these specimens, Nilsson made a deal with clinics in Stockholm and Gothenburg to take aborted and miscarried foetuses to his studio for use in his photo essay.

Using dead foetuses allowed Nilsson to set the stage with lighting and positioning to place a foetus's thumb in its mouth. He didn't have long before the specimens started to degenerate; keeping them in water helped, as did other tricks – fixing them in formaldehyde, coating them with a layer of gold, freezing them with liquid nitrogen – to create his story of growth and potential.

Following Nilsson's essay, ultrasound scanning became more routine. 3D imaging was possible from 1984 in Japan, and more widely from the 1990s, making it possible to see ever-more-naturalistic close-ups of a foetal face. In medical terms this is broadly positive, for it allows early detection of development problems, though there may not be solutions.

Many prospective parents swap notes in the global online villages of BabyCenter and Mumsnet. On community.babycenter.com, one woman reported that her first baby had been born 'with a severe cleft lip, cleft palate and microtia (deformed ear). She is now a beautiful, healthy almost 3 and a half years old! To me she is beautiful today (after her lip and palate repair) and was beautiful then . . . Now I am 30 weeks pregnant with my second child, we gone the u/s down [sic], our only concern was to have a healthy baby, so when the tech showed me his face, I was so grateful.'

What happens when the news isn't so positive? Medical ethics often play catch-up with medical innovations. Scans raise ethical issues about which foetuses are 'viable' and which should continue; globally that decision has meant discrimination against girls. In 1990, under the one-child policy that existed between 1980 and 2016, the Anhui province in eastern China banned ultrasound scanning; its use led to the disproportionate abortion of girls.

Beyond gender, scanning technologies open the door to eugenics, which we saw originated in the nineteenth century with Francis Galton, and the desire selectively to breed the best humans. What counts as undesirable? Should we be scanning for blindness? Deafness? Ugliness? Where do we draw the lines between what is an acceptable or an unacceptable 'disability'? And if anomalies are detected, how severe does a difference need to be for a foetus to be aborted?

In the case of Down's Syndrome, named after the English physician John Langdon Down, an extra chromosome produces a genetic disorder. People with Down's have developmental delays and a characteristic face: a flattened face, especially the bridge of the nose, almond-shaped, slanted eyes, and a tongue that tends to stick out. The risk of Down's increases in older mothers; in the U.K. scanning and amniotic sampling are routinely offered. But sampling, which is done through a needle via the abdominal wall, presents risks too. And around 90 per cent of positive results lead to abortion. The charity 'Don't Screen Us Out' argues that this high percentage is the result of legal and social discrimination, and fear.

Today, gene-editing technologies such as CRISPR, which has been used to target HPV genes E7 and E9 in cell lines, could help eliminate diseases that are carried genetically. In theory, the technologies could also be used to eliminate red hair or brown eyes, since these are also genetically inherited characteristics, or to create beautiful people who would benefit from social privilege. Obvious ethical problems arise: such as who decides what a perfect face looks like, and what kinds of inequities would we create?

This is more than a thought experiment. Although the world's population is unlikely to morph into Bella Hadid, there are many drawbacks to the idea of foetal scanning as a consumer choice. In the past, women imagined what their offspring would look like without any of the visual technologies we use today. They might principally have been concerned with whether they and their baby would survive the ordeal of birth, its health, and its sex. What a baby's face looked like, barring disability, would probably not have been high on the list of concerns.

The Face

That is not the case in the digital age. Today, an expectant parent can, for a price, access private 3D and even 4D scans (which include movement) to see what a foetus looks like. Initially used as enhanced medical scans, these have become 'photo opportunities' for the unwitting foetus. At 4dbabyscanslondon.com, customers are invited to connect with 'your yet to be born baby as we take a peek into the baby's world, see the face, hands, feet and sometimes, if lucky, see them yawn, wave or even smile'. In the same way that zookeepers recommend visiting chimps at feeding time, women attending scans are advised to eat sugary snacks to help 'keep the baby active and "posing for pictures" better'.

Expectant mothers might take up this opportunity, if they can afford the £500–£1,000 price tag, not only for reassurance, but also because it is sold as a bonding opportunity. Yet 3D and 4D scanning can have unintended consequences. On websites where pregnant women share concerns, they worry about having an ugly child. Take the woman who had a 4D ultrasound in 2012 and took to community.babycenter.com to complain that things hadn't gone as planned. 'My baby didn't look anything what I thought she would. She looked ugly with a big nose':

> Don't get me wrong, I will love my baby girl no matter what she looks like. I just was shocked that she looked the way she did. I never would have thought I'd be so vain to think my child was ugly and feel like a horrible mother for even thinking that.

Another user fretted 'my little girl looked like she had a huge nose in a couple shots, and we were totally freaked. Another shot it looked better, but I have this huge fear she will have a big nose. I have even debated getting another 3D because that was at 26 weeks. The wait is going to kill me. 8 weeks seems like so long!!!'

It's clear that scanning technologies set up several unrealistic expectations for expectant mothers, including what newborns will look like. The journey through the birth canal can be physically traumatic for babies as well as mothers, and newborn faces can be bruised and swollen for weeks. In the womb, too, foetal faces are squished and contorted; few are picture-perfect.

Some parents worry even after birth that their children – usually daughters – are going to find their looks a disadvantage. One Mumsnet user posted in 2023 that she had 'been to a lot of different baby groups with her, and I honestly find 99% of the babies there cute, except for mine . . . She's pale, has really small eyes, a huge nose and quite droopy features, so I worry these aren't things that will drastically improve.' Some respondents sympathized; others shared stories of their own ugly daughters; one recommended that the mother teach her child (who was still young enough to attend baby group) about cosmetics.

Judging foetuses and infants for how they look is an interesting, if depressing, extension of our interest in the foetal face. Some researchers argue that babies judge us too; eye-tracking studies suggest they prefer beautiful to ugly, and smiley to grumpy faces. In addition to the 'face hunger' babies display, as they search out faces as soon as they are born, foetuses are said to notice light patterns detectable through the mother's abdomen – especially if they resemble faces. Two eyes, a nose and a mouth arranged in lights capture the foetal gaze for longer than that same pattern of lights turned upside down, researchers at Lancaster University suggest.

It's reasonable to think babies have a neurological preference for faces, given we are inherently social beings. It is also likely that babies are more drawn to smiley faces than to grumpy ones, since those people are more likely to keep us safe. Most of our learning about others takes place in early infancy, but it makes sense that some cognitive hard wiring for pattern recognition exists in a foetal brain.

That pattern recognition does not, however, stretch to the Other Race Effect (ORE). This is the psychological phenomenon by which people are said to be better at recognizing other faces from the same ethnic or racial group.

But what do we mean by race? As the Human Genome Project proved from the 2010s, there are no individual 'races' that are genetically different; there is more genetic variation in a single population subgroup than between two different population subgroups.

The idea of one group of people being genetically different (let alone superior) to another, as the Victorians believed, is demonstrably false. Yes, different people exhibit specific features that reveal their geographic ancestry, but that's not the same thing as race. When we talk about race and ethnicity, we're really talking about perceived biological and cultural differences, as shaped by social and legal practices.

To give an example, Black babies are more likely to develop Sickle Cell Disease (SCD) than white babies, but not because all Black people carry it; about eight per cent have the trait that can lead to SCD, as their ancestors came from regions where it evolved to protect against malaria. That's a geographic rather than a racial distinction.

African American babies are twice as likely to die in their first year than non-Hispanic and Euro-American babies. This is because social and economic habits mean that African Americans have poorer living standards and are treated differently by medical systems. Sometimes what looks like a biological difference is a cultural one.

Which brings us back to the faces of foetuses and babies. There is no genetic reason why a white newborn baby might prefer white faces to Black or vice versa. The ORE has been used as evidence of some inherent racial bias. Which is nonsense – it appears only at the age of six months or so, when babies' perceptual world begins to narrow. That means they become more 'fine-tuned' visually to the things and people they see regularly. If the people they see are mostly Black, or white, then they will be better at recognizing that group of people. A 'mixed race' child is less likely to experience ORE, if they mix with people from a wider group.

So, babies aren't racist. Foetal scanning, however, can be. As we have seen throughout this book, all technologies are designed and used by people with their own in-built biases. Without consciousness of that bias we can make presumptions that don't stand up to scrutiny.

Take foetal alcohol syndrome. We know that excessive alcohol consumption by a pregnant mother affects the face of a foetus. A child with foetal alcohol syndrome typically has smaller eyes, a lower nasal bridge, a thinner upper lip and a philtrum that is smoother, and 0.4 mm longer than 'typical'. Foetal face measurements using 3D scanners allow clinicians to make those small, precise measurements, if the foetus doesn't move too much. But the algorithms used to determine foetal alcohol syndrome are not objective.

The Lancet medical journal declared in 1998 that 'tough measures' were needed to address maternal alcohol consumption in South Africa, since foetuses in the Western Cape had the highest incidence of foetal alcohol syndrome in the world. The moralizing language around alcohol consumption in pregnancy originated in the late 1970s. The timing is interesting since this was a critical moment in the second wave of feminism. Historically, attempts to control women's bodies have taken place when patriarchy is challenged. We can see the U.S. overturning of abortion rights with *Roe v. Wade* (2022) as a patriarchal response to the #MeToo movement.

Now, it is true that the Western Cape has a heavy-drinking culture, largely because of the 'dop system' introduced by seventeenth-century Europeans into South Africa. Under the system farm workers received part of their wages in alcohol, which led to widespread alcoholism, especially among the 'Cape Coloured' community, that is, South Africans with a wide variety of ethnic backgrounds – Dutch, African Xhosa, Khoisan, German, Irish, Indian, French, Malaysian and British ancestry.

However, there is more to these findings than meets the eye. A depressed nasal bridge, thinner upper lip or longer philtrum are not always signs of a clinical disorder; sometimes they are healthy ethnic variants. In Cape Coloured foetal scans, all false negatives came from white Finnish populations. A parallel study of Down's syndrome in Congolese and Belgian populations found that Belgian samples were 80 per cent accurate, whereas Congolese samples were only 35 per cent accurate.

What does this mean for healthcare equity, and how we read a foetal face? There is an acknowledged healthcare disparity in the U.K. and the U.S. with poorer maternal and infant health outcomes for Black populations when compared to white ones. Changing that means addressing where racism has infiltrated science.

We should not be relying on screening tests without using a properly inclusive data set. In the U.S., African American children are far more likely to be diagnosed with foetal alcohol syndrome than white children. This is also true of the native Inuit population in Saskatchewan, Canada, for whom there are no established norms, and children normally have a nasal bridge depression. Yet aboriginal mothers who drink any alcohol at all while pregnant with their children routinely receive a diagnosis of foetal alcohol syndrome.

In Barcelona, the Baby Face Model (BFM) was developed by scientists to compare ultrasound images with postnatal images, to discover how reliable those ultrasound scans are. Although the BFM was intended to address all ethnic groups, nearly half of all data used was taken from white faces, and only a quarter from Black faces. As a result, if a scanned foetus had lips bigger than the norms imposed, the scanner presumed its mouth was open. Given the current healthcare crises in the U.K. and the U.S. over poorer maternal health outcomes in Black communities, we need to rethink how we look at foetal faces.

It is striking that in just over sixty years since Lennart Nilsson's famous image of a child *in utero* on the cover of *Life* magazine, clinical and media images of foetuses and babies remain overwhelmingly white. This discrepancy was noted by Chidiebere Ibe, a Nigerian medical illustrator, when he was a medical student in Zambia. Having lost his mother to fibroid surgery, Ibe became an advocate for improvements in maternal and antenatal care. In 2020, having found that fewer than 5 per cent of medical images show dark skin, Ibe began drawing medical illustrations with Black people as his subjects.

In 2021, Ibe went viral on social media with his illustration of a foetus in the womb – the first ever medical representation of a Black child *in utero* (fig. 24). This artwork has had a profound cultural

Grown

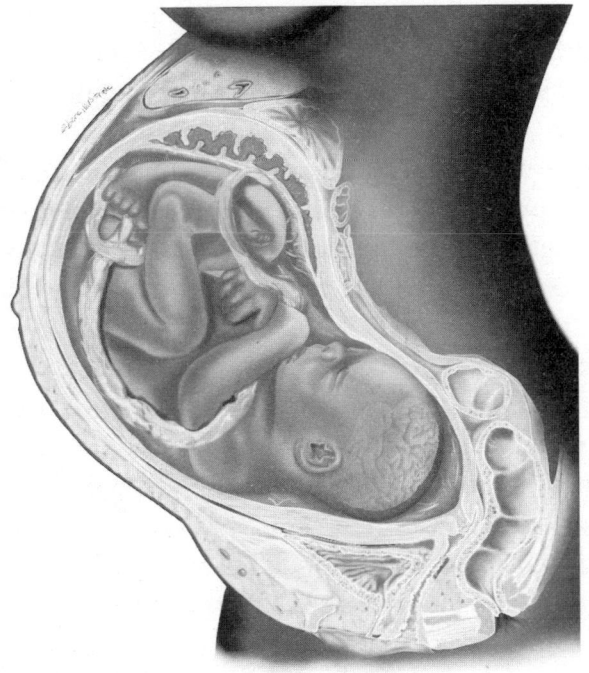

24. Chidiebere Ibe, a Black child *in utero*, 2021.

impact, and Ibe has since collaborated with Johnson & Johnson and Deloitte Digital to produce a digital library of diverse medical images: illustratechange.com. The site shows how differently symptoms appear according to skin colour; one example is cyanosis, a bluish-purple colour of the skin that is most easily seen where the skin is thin – on the lips, mouth, earlobes and fingernails. Cyanosis indicates insufficient oxygen in the bloodstream but may be overlooked if clinicians use data drawn from white bodies.

What can we learn from this moment in history, and from the scanning of infant and baby faces? Medical technologies have created the womb as a place accessible to outsiders, which at the same time confirms the public status of the foetus: individuated and separated from its mother, long before it could survive independently. How we interpret the face of a foetus, what we consider normal or abnormal development, and whose faces we choose to represent in textbooks all reflect deeper assumptions about human worth and belonging. As we move forward into an era of even more sophisticated foetal imaging and genetic editing technologies, understanding this history becomes more crucial than ever.

Humans are apparently programmed to find foetal and baby faces particularly appealing. This results from a 'baby schema' (*Kindchenschema*) identified by the Austrian zoologist Konrad Lorenz; infants have characteristics that we are evolutionarily destined to find cute – a large head, round face and big eyes – so that we will take care of them.

And yet there must be more to it than that, since we do not universally care for babies and children; refugee children, or those living in war zones, do not benefit widely from our compassion or care. It is worth noting that Lorenz himself was a member of the Nazi Party and joked about Jews, though he later said he regretted that.

Knowing what a foetus looked like, and being able to represent that face to others, has been a critical step in giving the foetus rights, ethical or otherwise. And that reveals something important about the history of the face more generally; to be given personhood, to receive empathy, we need to have a face. This is not a passive face, or an indifferent face, but a feeling face, meaning one that we can invest with meanings and emotions. That is a fundamental part of being human, after all.

But how do we know how to read faces? And what happens when we don't, or can't, express how we feel? We will find out in the following chapter.

6.
Expressed

When Kathleen Bogart was born, the delivery room fell into an unexpected quiet; there was no grimace or flicker of expression on her face, and no lusty cry of indignation. The attending physician frowned and noted her stillness on her hospital chart. Within hours, he had delivered his verdict: failure to thrive. This was a generic term still in use in 1981, when Kathleen came into the world in an American hospital. Newborns without facial expressions were presumed to have severe cognitive impairment, even brain damage. A baby who couldn't cry must be fundamentally lacking in human potential. The best thing for it, the doctor told Kathleen's parents, was to place their child in an institution.

Fortunately, her parents did not listen to the physician. For the next two years they sought a better understanding of Kathleen's condition, consulting specialist after specialist until she was finally diagnosed with Moebius syndrome – a rare syndrome that affects one in 50,000 infants a year in the U.S. It is caused by the underdevelopment of the facial nerves I discussed in the previous chapter; those nerves activate our facial muscles and allow us to frown, laugh and cry as well as smile, all of which are important for emotional communication.

Moebius syndrome is not the only health condition that causes facial paralysis – Bell's palsy is the most common, affecting 40,000 people a year in the U.S.; other causes include Ramsay Hunt syndrome (famously experienced by the pop star Justin Bieber), traumatic injuries, viruses, surgeries and strokes.

Kathleen has not only thrived, she has achieved considerable success, and helped many other people with facial paralysis along the way; she is now Professor of Psychology and Director of the Disability and Social Interaction Laboratory at Oregon State University. She is also a Fellow of the Society for Personality and Social Psychology, and an advocate for people with rare disorders, including Moebius syndrome.

What, then, are we to make of the reaction of Kathleen's attending physician? It was surprisingly common, even in the late-twentieth century for parents to be 'relieved' of the burden of caring for a child with disabilities. And presuming a child without facial expression to be lacking in thought and emotion is also still common. For centuries, facial expression has been used alongside language to separate humans from 'lesser' animals; the more complex the repertoire of expressions, it has been presumed, the more evolved the being. And humans have a much wider range of expressions than any other animal.

Many species do show emotions through their faces. Most primates – chimpanzees, gorillas and orangutans – have a fear grimace and a play face. Dogs have 'puppy dog' eyes or a 'hangdog' expression when sad; they also curl their lips to show aggression and seem to smile when happy. Elephants, horses, birds and rats also use some variation of expression that involves their eyes, mouths and ears. There are differences of opinion about what those expressions mean. Is it sentimental to believe that animals – especially our domesticated pets – feel emotions as profoundly as humans?

The answer depends on how we value animals – and which ones. In ancient Rome the physician Galen taught students about the body by vivisection, that is, cutting animals up alive – pigs, sheep, goats, monkeys, birds and lions. William Harvey also vivisected animals in the seventeenth century to demonstrate the circulation of the blood.

Neither man thought he was being cruel; they simply didn't believe animals had souls, or feelings. And the two things – souls and feelings – were connected; 'passions' were believed to be the spirit moving through the body, in the pursuit of good and avoidance of evil. By contrast, the expressions of pain or fear showed by animals under the knife, vivisectionists believed, were reflex physical reactions: they had no emotional meaning. The same logic would later be applied to humans deemed 'lesser': enslaved people, colonized populations, people with disabilities.

By the eighteenth century, moral sensibility around vivisection was changing. 'The question is not, Can [animals] *reason*? nor, Can they *talk*? but, Can they *suffer*?' wrote the philosopher Jeremy Bentham. For the philosopher, the morality of an action was determined by the degree of pleasure or pain it generated.

Vivisection did not stop; it peaked in the nineteenth century with the work of the French physiologist Claude Bernard. But the growing sensibility around animal suffering gave rise to protective societies, such as the Royal Society for the Prevention of Cruelty to Animals (RSPCA). Vivisection was regulated by the U.K.'s Cruelty to Animals Act (1876); there was no comparable ban in the U.S. – instead the Animal Welfare Act (1966) established guidelines. Individual states still decide what is acceptable and what is not.

This heightened, outward sensibility is characteristic of modern Western emotional standards; it is no longer acceptable to mistreat animals, or to hang and flog people in public. We are more sensitive to the suffering of animals, and in part this reflects an awareness that they feel, though speciesism means we care more about dogs and cats than cows and rats.

Human expression is also more sophisticated than that of animals for reasons of anatomy – which gives a clue to the face's function, and our unique social organization. We have around forty-three facial muscles (depending on how you count); monkeys and chimps have twenty-three. This difference allows humans to have far more complex and subtle expressions. Some muscles are specialized for very fine movements, what psychologists call micro-expressions, in the subtle signs of the eyes, eyebrows, mouth and cheeks. Those muscles are also part of a feedback loop, which means that smiling can make us happier, while frowning makes us grumpier.

That feedback loop raises questions about the use of Botox, and whether it can impact on what emotions we feel as well as express.

Some studies argue that if we can't smile, we can't feel happy, but Kathleen and others would disagree! People with paralysis feel emotions, though that feeling might be less visible.

There is an interesting parallel in display codes between Western and Eastern cultures; Japanese people are less demonstrative than American people, though that doesn't mean they feel less deeply. In Japan, emotional display is governed by the concept of 'wa' (和), which literally means harmony. Since Japan is more collectivist than the U.S., hiding certain feelings is necessary to show respect and to protect *wa*. By contrast, American culture has a high level of individualism, and emotional displays are demonstrative; service workers are trained to be smiley and happy and even fawning, though this can seem fake to tourists. Americans criticize the emotional reserve of Japanese people as aloofness, or, with all its racist undertones, inscrutability.

In Japan, the concept of 'face', referred to as 'mentsu' (面子), is more complex than in the U.S.; it signifies not only a person's appearance, but also their public image and social standing. Avoiding situations that could cause people to 'lose face' is far more important in the East than in the West because of the way in which social harmony is core to one's sense of self and position in society. To lose face or honour can mean a loss of one's identity, relationship or job. In the U.S., it tends to mean a temporary social embarrassment.

These diverse contexts matter if we want to understand the trajectory of emotional expressions – and what they mean – in the West, which is the focus of this book. We have seen that many European ideas and beliefs were passed down by ancient Greek theorists like Aristotle. He also influenced the teachings of St Jerome, who translated the first Bible in Latin, known as the Vulgate, in the late fourth century.

St Jerome was known for his deep reflections on the human soul, virtue and morality. 'The face is the mirror of the mind,' he famously said, 'and eyes without speaking confess the secrets of the heart.' We saw how this belief, that the essence of the self was conveyed in the face, was developed in portraiture from the Renaissance.

Expressed

Portraiture is static of course, unlike emotional expression. It is one thing to convey a person's character in the shape of a nose, or the squaring of a chin, but quite another in the curling of a lip or the furrow of a brow. In the eighteenth century, pathognomy became a separate field that was added to physiognomy (largely due to the work of Lavater, whom we met in an earlier chapter).

By studying the movement of the face, pathognomists believed they could predict exactly what a person was thinking or feeling. And we still believe that. We see it in medicine, when healthcare professionals use facial expressions to determine a person's pain, discomfort or emotional state, and in policing, as officers watch for facial signs of fear or nervousness and determine if a person looks 'shifty'. In marketing, facial-recognition cameras track and analyse consumers' expressions when they view advertisements and products, to determine whether people want to buy (or steal) certain goods.

And we do it all the time in our personal and professional lives – we hire people with 'honest' facial expressions; we cross the road to avoid people based on a look; we decide whether to trust a person based on whether they seem 'off'. Some of this is intuition; our brains and bodies are interpreting hundreds of minute pieces of information at once, from a person's gesture and odour to their clothing, their tone of voice, their energy.

We attribute most of these feelings to a person's expression; a smiling face is read as an invitation to approach while a scowl keeps us away. Most of the time we don't consciously register that we are using expressions to judge a person's intelligence, just as Kathleen's doctors had done.

Where do we learn what these expressions mean? Again, there is an element of intuition – most of us can tell when a smile is fake, or there is a disconnect between what a person says and what their face does.

As with all other aspects of the face, there is also a rich history of writing in philosophy and medicine about what facial expressions mean – which can't be separated from how many emotions people believed to exist. Before we think about what emotional faces mean now, let's take a detour into the history of facial expression, because we will find the same threads – about categorization, hierarchies, truth and the need to know that recur repeatedly in the history of the face.

Aristotle thought there were seventeen emotional types, six of which were linked to pain and the remainder to pleasure. Both pain and pleasure were guided by the soul that separated humans from animals – in humoral theory, which dominated Western medicine from the second to the eighteenth centuries, emotional expressions were signs that the soul was moving towards something good or fleeing from something bad. So, in love and desire, the face flushed as the blood rushed towards the object of your affection, but in fear the soul retreated, making the face pale and the hair stand on end.

Black people couldn't have the kind of sensibility given to whites, because their cheeks did not pale, theorists reasoned; only white people were sophisticated enough to blush. This pseudoscience served colonial rulers and slave owners alike.

Emotion theory became more sophisticated from the Renaissance, though no less biased in favour of European experience, as we saw earlier in this book. The anatomical dissections of artists such as Leonardo da Vinci, and later of Andreas Vesalius – the anatomist whose beautifully illustrated work *On the Fabric of the Body in Seven Books* critiqued much of Galen's theories – allowed for a far more detailed understanding of the muscles and nerves of the face, and of expression. This shift allowed Renaissance artists to create ever more realistic and individualized portraits.

Emotional expression in painting was formalized in the seventeenth century by the French artist Charles Le Brun. He was incidentally the decorator of the Palace of Versailles, including its Hall of Mirrors, which we encountered in chapter three. Le Brun was also the First Painter to the King in Louis XIV's reign, and a founding member of the Royal Academy of Painting and Sculpture.

In 1668 Le Brun presented a lecture to the Royal Academy on how to depict human emotions accurately. The lecture was given because the Royal Academy wanted a set of principles for the painter's practice that could demonstrate 'an academic science of painting'.

Where did this desire come from? Today it's unfashionable to talk about a 'scientific revolution' – that's because all revolutions are evolutions if you dig deep enough. (We no longer talk about industrial revolution in the nineteenth century either, seeing the origins of technological change as far back as the 1700s.) But the Renaissance spirit of inquiry and humanism was fertile ground for scientific discoveries; Copernicus's heliocentric model (depicting the sun as the centre of the universe) and Isaac Newton's discovery of gravity were both part of the humanistic inquiry explored earlier in this book.

Unsurprisingly, getting to grips with the relationship between mind and body was part of this rethinking of the fundamentals of human knowledge. The French philosopher René Descartes introduced the idea that mind and body were separate, now a fundamental premise of scientific medicine, in his 1641 book *Meditations on First Philosophy*.

Before this time, the mind and body had been imagined holistically, and according to the four humours discussed in chapter two. Descartes argued that the mind (or *psyche*, which also meant soul) was separate from the body; the mind was an immaterial, thinking substance, but the body was a material and instinctual one. This made it easier for people to think about the body as a machine that operated independently, while the essence of thought was in the mind. Descartes summed this up in his famous statement 'Cogito, ergo sum' ('I think, therefore I am').

If mind and body were separate – the principle that became Cartesianism – then the kind of scientific inquiry laid down by the scientist Francis Bacon, ordered, rational and unemotional, was entirely possible. That spirit of empirical, reasoned research was the context of Carl Linnaeus's ordering of humans by appearance, as explored in chapter two, and subsequent Victorian hierarchies of people and things.

So it made sense for Le Brun and later writers that art and depictions of the face could be governed by the same basic ordering principle as everything else. If the French Royal Academy could determine an academic science of beauty, that would also help ennoble art as a scientific practice at a time when artists were being celebrated as never before. Portraiture might only have been categorized as the second most important type of painting – the first being history painting, meaning great mythical, allegorical and historical studies – but standardizing a painterly code for emotions would help formalize teaching.

Le Brun leaned into the work of his compatriot in putting this together, especially Descartes' *Les Passions de l'âme* (*The Passions of the Soul*), published in 1649. In this work, Descartes expanded on the ideas of his *Meditations* and argued that emotional expressions were proof that the mind worked in and through the physical body. Descartes did not include much detail about this, or any images, which is where Le Brun saw the value he could bring.

Published posthumously in 1698 as *Méthode pour apprendre à dessiner les passions* (*Method for Learning to Draw the Passions*), Le Brun's work depicted Descartes' six core passions in twenty-three 'expressive heads': admiration or wonder, love, hate, desire, joy and sadness. Le Brun also included others, such as compassion, scorn and laughter (fig. 25). In laughter, he wrote, which was caused by joy and surprise:

> the eyebrows rise towards the middle of the eye, and bend towards the sides of the nose; the eyes are almost shut and sometimes appear half wet, or shed tears, which make no alteration in the face; the mouth, half open, shows the teeth; the corners of the mouth drawn back, cause a wrinkle in the cheeks, which appear so swelled as to hide the eyes in some measure; the nostrils are open, and all the face is of a red colour.

If you had to describe what happened when someone laughed, could you do any better? Notice, though, that Le Brun does not mention the anatomy of the face, and his description is a caricature – like his sketches. They show generically white and mostly male figures, especially when strong and intense emotions like rage or terror are depicted. Softer, more feminine faces were used to illustrate melancholy or sadness.

Expressed

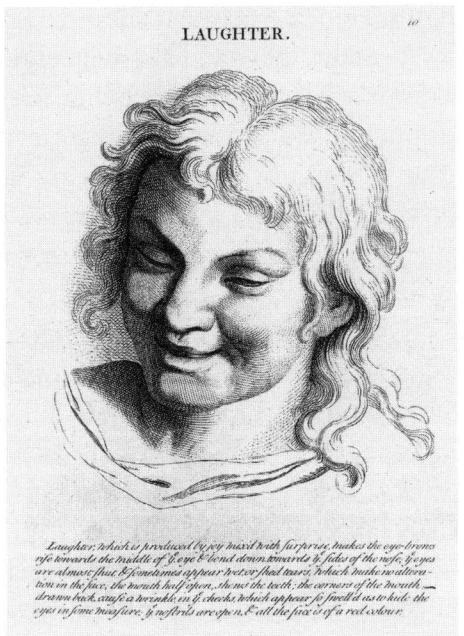

25. 'Laughter' Plate 10, Charles Le Brun, 1760.

This gendering echoed Galenic beliefs that men were angrier than women because their bodies were hotter – in men, excess humours were burned up; in women, they led to menstruation and weeping.

For Le Brun, as for Descartes, the eyes were particularly expressive because the soul sat in the pineal gland, just behind the eyes; this explains why eyebrows were particularly expressive. Incidentally, this belief about the soul has resonance in Hinduism, and the so-called 'third eye' – associated with intuition, mysticism and insight; as with Buddhism, Hinduism locates the third eye in the middle of the forehead.

Le Brun's work was hugely popular in Europe. By the mid-1700s, the *Method* had been translated into English, Italian, and German. For the first time, artists across Europe were working from the same emotional playbook, which helps to explain the focus on subjective experience discussed in the chapter on portraiture.

By the 1800s, the idea of the soul would shift, and with it, the idea of emotional expression. The Scottish surgeon and anatomist Sir Charles Bell (coincidentally, the man who first described Bell's palsy) published several books about the human body based on his dissections. He was less interested in the soul than in the musculature and focused on the function of the face. His work was influenced by religion; he believed that only humans had the musculature for a wide range of emotional expressions because they had a special relationship with God.

But predictably, given all we have learned about scientific bias, not all humans were considered equal. Distinguishing between humans in the same prejudiced way that Linnaeus had, Bell noted the 'peculiarities in the head of the negro and Calmuc [Mongolian]'; seeing a hierarchy of faces that demonstrate the supremacy of whites: 'the appearance of the head passes from that of the European to that of the negro – from that of the negro, to that of the brute'.

Bell's work on the face influenced Charles Darwin's *The Expression of the Emotions in Man and Animals* (1872). Darwin did not believe in physiognomy; he had in fact been judged unfairly himself as lacking in the face department. When he tried to join the HMS *Beagle*, the ship on which he sailed to the Galapagos Islands (1831–6), he was originally denied entry because its captain, Robert FitzRoy, felt that no man with a nose like Darwin's had the energy and the determination for such a voyage.

Despite this inauspicious start Darwin persuaded the captain of his worth, and on that voyage became especially interested in the theme of emotions. He was fascinated by the behaviours of the peoples of Tierra del Fuego, an archipelago at the southern tip of South America, and began noting the facial and bodily expressions of humans and animals in his notebooks. He also studied his infant son Doddy (whom we met in the chapter on mirrors), and experimented by raising his voice to him, poking and tickling him; at other times Darwin roared in anger and withheld affection, just to see how Doddy responded.

Darwin's research on emotions was only possible through the medium of photography. Victorian scientists were great correspondents, and Darwin used his networks to collect photographs of infants from friends and fellow researchers; he also acquired photographs of patients in asylums from James Crichton-Browne, a psychiatrist at Yorkshire's West Riding Lunatic Asylum. Darwin placed these images alongside ethnographic photographs to capture and compare specific emotions as if they were specimens from natural history.

However, as we saw in the chapter on photography, the early technology was frustrating – it was light dependent, and even then, the exposure times could be too long to capture the fleeting grimace or frown. So, Darwin commissioned the photographer Oscar Rejlander, best known for his montage prints and sentimental images of children, to create a series of images for his *Expression of the Emotions in Man and Animals*. This couldn't be done in the winter, because of the lack of natural light, but by the following spring Rejlander obliged.

Rejlander was used to working with theatrical performers to create his images, and he wasn't averse to standing before the camera himself – including to show the expression labelled 'contempt' (fig. 26). The images he sold Darwin included that of a crying baby, which went on to sell commercially as a stand-alone

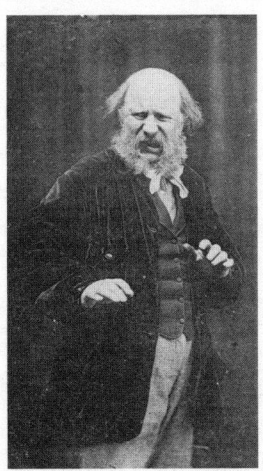

26. Oscar Rejlander, 'Contempt', in Charles Darwin's *The Expression of the Emotions in Man and Animals*, 1872.

image (named after an unfortunate character in a literary satire, the print became known as 'Ginx's Baby').

Darwin sent copies of his images to collaborators around the world, asking them what mood was displayed by a particular image of someone laughing or frowning or looking scornful. All of this was intended to establish a universal measure of emotion. As we will see, this is broadly the same methodology used in emotion theory today.

Darwin received thirty-six replies to his questionnaire, which seems an incredibly small number given what came next; he used that data, along with his own analyses, to conclude that human facial expression emerged by evolution and adaptation. Some expressions, like the baring of teeth in anger, he explained as a vestige from the way we used teeth – as animals do – rather than weapons, to fight.

The fact that teeth-baring is a universally understood anger-display in primates, Darwin concluded, showed that humans and animals shared a common inheritance. Similarly, crying was a form of communication that pre-dated language; before children learn to speak, they make crying and screaming sounds as notes in a musical scale, rather like gibbons. And Darwin noted that all infants cried alike – and with the same expression as Ginx's Baby. His description is reminiscent of Le Brun's account of laughter:

> their eyes are firmly closed, so that the skin round them is wrinkled, and the forehead contracted into a frown. The mouth is widely opened with the lips retracted in a peculiar manner, which causes it to assume a squarish form; the gums or teeth being more or less exposed.

Darwin found plenty of infants screaming that he could observe, but he wanted photographs because then he could really study the face in detail.

While Darwin commissioned photographs from the theatrically minded Rejlander, the French physiologist Guillaume Duchenne de Boulogne found another solution to the problem of rapid expressions against slow exposure times. He experimented with 'electropuncture' – that is, administering electric shocks to people's faces to make the muscles contract and 'fix' the expression. Then he took photographs, which he published in *Mécanisme de la physionomie humaine* (*The Mechanism of Human Facial Expression*, 1862).

Duchenne subjected the faces of six people to this treatment, only one of whom was not his patient, which raises ethical questions for the modern viewer. One of his most frequently used subjects was an 'old toothless man, with a thin face, whose features, without being absolutely ugly, approached ordinary triviality' (fig. 27).

Duchenne was particularly interested in using this anonymous old man for his experiments because his face, lacking teeth, had less resistance around the mouth; his absence of facial hair also made it easier for Duchenne to show the effects of stimulating different muscle groups. Nobody thought about the impact on the old man.

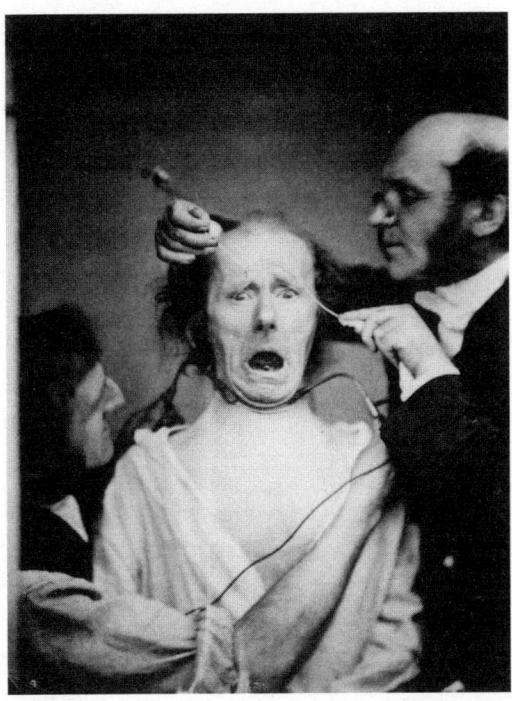

27. Guillaume Duchenne and 'the old toothless man', 1862.

Darwin and Duchenne's interest in facial expression paralleled the measuring, recording and comparing of the face that we discussed in other chapters – from portraiture to mugshots. Darwin's *Expression* was published as a kind of sequel to *On the Origin of Species* (1859) and *The Descent of Man* (1871); *Origin* explained evolution, *Descent* discussed how humans are related to other species, and *Expression* focused on how humans used their faces to survive and communicate.

Although it's not as well known as Darwin's other works, *Expression* was read widely – it also influenced broader theories about what it was to be human in the sciences of the mind, which originated in the same period. Sigmund Freud's work on hysteria referenced Darwin when describing emotional expressions as 'actions which originally had a meaning and served a purpose'. While the psychologist and philosopher William James developed Darwin's work on the physical dimensions of emotion, as we will see shortly.

In the twentieth century, interest in expression shifted to the question of universalism, rather than evolution. In Darwin's work universalism was determined by the consensus reached by people he consulted about what emotional faces meant. But as we saw, Darwin's conclusions were based on limited data, and early anthropology used methods and ideas that are no longer culturally acceptable.

The German-American anthropologist Franz Boas argued that evolution was used to support ethnocentrism, the idea that Western people were superior to so-called 'primitive' cultures. He argued in favour of relativism; the idea that each culture was unique and should be studied on its own terms. Boas didn't specifically focus on emotional expression, but he did challenge the biological simplicity of Darwin's ideas. Boas's student Margaret Mead undertook fieldwork in Samoa, examining how cultures affected adolescent behaviour and emotional development.

Mead has since been criticized for misunderstanding Samoan culture, but her findings confirmed that emotional patterns and expressions were learned and not purely biological. Of course, this was a threat to Darwin's model; Darwin believed that emotions were adaptive and deeply rooted in evolution, whereas Mead thought they could be reshaped or eliminated by habit.

I am oversimplifying slightly to highlight the gap between biological versus cultural approaches, a subject that has fuelled much discussion about nature and nurture ever since. A reasonable approach, as we will see, is some sort of middle ground – we have the capacity to make a wide range of emotional expressions, some of which are no longer useful, but we are nevertheless influenced by culture. One need only observe a Japanese person arguing with an Italian, or a British person with an American, to see the weight of culture first hand.

Yet we still see emotional expressions as primarily biological – partly because of the influence of Darwin, and partly because of the work of Paul Ekman, who is probably the most famous psychologist working on human emotions. As a psychologist, Ekman looks for universal human patterns, which favours a biological approach; as an anthropologist, Mead focuses on cultural variation and the influence of social learning.

At a disciplinary level, then, Ekman and Mead were predisposed to disagree. Mead criticized Ekman's work on the universality of emotional expression; his subjects were too influenced by Western culture, she said, and the faces they had seen in movies and magazines.

In response, Ekman went to Papua New Guinea, to find the most isolated people he could – the Fore tribe; they had no knowledge of Western culture, and therefore could not have been influenced by its emotional repertoire. There he undertook a series of tests that used Darwin's basic methodology; showing the faces of emotional people to non-Western subjects and asking them what was being expressed.

The way he worked was this: Ekman and his researcher told members of the tribe a story and asked them to choose which emotion was most appropriate for that story from a range of photographs. If the story was about a man who was happy, for instance, then the subjects would be asked to choose between a sad face, a disgusted face and a happy face. Ekman concluded that since members of the Fore tribe always picked the same face as his Western subjects did, emotional expressions were universal, implicating the amygdala.

Except there was some criticism of Ekman's methods, including the suggestion that he bribed participants with cigarettes and soap. Even without that there was ample scope for persuasion; how a researcher *told* a story would surely influence the reaction of listeners – you can make a story sound light or sad or repulsive depending on your tone of voice.

From his findings, however, Ekman compiled a list of six basic emotions – anger, disgust, happiness, sadness, fear and surprise. Later he would add contempt, the emotion that Rejlander had acted out for Darwin; Ekman did not initially include this, as he worried it wasn't so easy to detect as an emotional expression.

Ekman used that list to build a map of facial expressions, just as Duchenne had done, but without inserting electrodes into the face of an old, toothless man. Emotional expressions are 'involuntary', he insisted – they 'appear even when we don't want them to'. There might be 'display rules' that determined whether they were shown, he said in a concession to Mead, but still the hidden signs of emotion were there, if we knew how to read them.

That led to Ekman's claims about 'micro-expressions', and the belief that the face can 'lie and tell the truth and often does both at the same time'. He set out those tell-tale clues in his book *Telling Lies: Clues to Deceit in the Marketplace, Politics and Marriage* (1985). Most people, the book claims, don't know how to read between the lines, and tell when a person is lying – he could help them learn.

Whatever else, Ekman is a terrific salesman; he set out a system called the Facial Action Coding System (FACS) that is said to allow the 'objective' measurement of facial movements. Based on that work, he has secured several prestigious advisory roles, in marketing, law enforcement and artificial intelligence (AI). His work is used by computer animators to create realistic cartoon faces for films such as *Inside Out* (Pixar, 2015) and by the U.S. Department of

Homeland Security to train staff to identify potential hijackers. He was also involved in the popular TV show *Lie to Me* (20th Century Fox Television, 2009–11), one of many programmes that presumes facial expressions are universal and lies detectable – if only you can crack the code.

The convenience of the model is key; who doesn't want to believe they can read infidelity in their lover's smirk or anticipate whether their boss is about to fire them?

What we see time and again in the history of facial expression is attempts to formalize, classify and explain the emotions of others – something that has become ever more important in the centuries since Le Brun – for politics and trade, to navigate busy social and urban environments, for safety, policing and education, to support all the social systems and networks that went into a modern bureaucratic environment.

Kathleen Bogart's story illuminates perfectly the challenges of making such truth claims. Born into a world where her inability to make facial expressions was read as intellectual impairment, she now lives in an era where AI systems claim to read our emotions with mathematical precision. The irony is striking; we have moved from human doctors making devastating assumptions with medical certainty to computer algorithms that are equally certain – and equally wrong.

Take Microsoft's emotion-recognition software (Azure Face), which was designed in 2018 to recognize faces and emotions across different cultures. This system used Paul Ekman's seven core emotions to train Azure Face on large data sets of facial images that were then analysed for patterns that match emotional expression.

Other direct links with Ekman's research have been made by Affectiva (now part of the Swedish company Smart Eye), which uses computer-vision and deep-learning algorithms to analyse facial expressions for advertising research; Realeyes (the U.K. and Hungary), which tracks emotional responses in marketing and advertising; and Face++ (China), part of the TimeSense group, a leader in AI.

Are emotional expressions *really* that simple, that they can be used and reused, analysed and copied regardless of cultural context? Historians of emotion, like anthropologists, have been saying no to this for decades. Mostly, historians critique display codes, like Ekman's, but some of us feel that emotions, too, are culturally constructed. I have argued this most clearly about loneliness, as a particular emotion that we consider universal and individual, but is historically specific, with social and economic causes.

More recently, neuroscientists have focused on the cultural; their research tends to attract more attention than that of scholars in the humanities – probably because of the weight Western culture gives to brain scans as a form of objective evidence. I will come back to brain scans in chapter eight.

Lisa Feldman Barrett's work bridges neuroscience and psychology. She has written several influential books about how emotions work in the mind and the body, using functional magnetic resonance imaging (fMRI) scanning to observe how neural changes correspond to reported emotions.

Barrett has also worked outside the laboratory; while Ekman studied isolated people in Papua New Guinea, she did fieldwork with the Himba – hunter-gatherers living in Namibia. She also asked them to sort through photographic images, using the same methodology as Darwin and Ekman, but her results were different; the Himba seem not to categorize facial expressions in the same way that Westerners do. They did not group faces showing wide-eyed, open-mouth expressions under the category of 'fear'. Their view of expressions was more action- and context-based – for example, a person looking at something, rather than expressing a single emotional state.

Barrett argues that emotions are culturally constructed in the following way – we learn emotions as concepts in our culture (remember how children like to pull faces in the mirror?), and we interpret the emotional world depending on our language and concepts. The brain then uses that emotional framing to make sense of our experience.

In some ways this is not a new finding – it takes us back to the psychologist and philosopher William James, who argued that emotions are felt in the body and then framed by the mind. In a famous article 'What is Mind?' written in 1899, James argued that we might see a bear in the woods, for instance, and have a physical reaction – and then our mind settles on an emotion that fits; fear if we are sensible. Similarly, 'we don't cry because we're sad,' he said, 'we're sad because we cry'.

Barrett's approach, though, is to take issue with other neuroscientists, and psychologists such as Ekman, who have oversimplified emotional expressions and emotions themselves; she argues against 'emotion circuits' or specific brain regions for fear or love or anger. She sees emotions as happenings or feelings that become 'emotions' because of our cultural frameworks.

This is more than saying that emotions are expressed differently in different cultures – which was Ekman's concession to Mead. We saw this earlier on when contrasting American ways of emoting with Japanese; we might similarly say that British people of a certain class have a 'stiff upper lip' mentality, which contrasts with the emotional openness found in Arabic communities.

Many cultures value displays of emotion even without the emotion – professional mourners were once common in Egyptian, Chinese, Mediterranean and Near Eastern cultures, in recognition of the social importance of tears. And all cultures have gendered display codes. However fluid we might see gender today in the West, it is still common to hear such phrases as 'boys don't cry'; emotions like fear and sadness are gendered female, whereas anger and pride are gendered male.

What Barrett, and some historians of emotion, say is more radical: it is not just the expression of emotions that are different but the emotions themselves. Facial expressions cannot be signals of pure emotion, then, as they are for Darwin or Ekman, because they are culturally sensitive signs that make sense within specific communities. We misread them when we bring our own bag of presumptions; when you have a hammer, everything looks like a nail.

Barrett found that when people are asked to freely label facial expressions (without using the constrained word lists given by Ekman as emotion categories) there is far more disagreement about what those expressions mean. And when the study was repeated with the Hazda people in Tanzania, people didn't label emotional expressions in the same way at all – suggesting that the consensus Ekman reported was a product of his methodology, rather than evidence of universal emotions.

It's also presumptuous to think that people in different cultures view the face in the same way. They don't – and that's one reason why mask-wearing caused so many complaints in the U.S. during the Covid-19 pandemic; this wasn't just about civil liberties, but a more fundamental issue about human communication. In the West, when we talk to people we focus more on the mouth, and that's where we look for clues to how a person really feels. In East Asia, the eyes are a more important aspect of emotional communication – partly because display codes are more subtle, but also because wearing masks in Japan and China has been common since the 1918 Spanish Flu pandemic.

As ever with the face, gender and race come into play too; Black people are less likely to be believed when they express pain and more likely to be seen as angry, because of the cultural stereotypes we saw in other chapters. Women are more likely to smile to appease a man, and to be told to 'cheer up', especially in the U.K.

What about mixed emotions – how can we pinpoint a single emotional state if a person feels anger and sadness at the same time? Some people have more malleable and expressive faces than others, and some conditions, such as Parkinson's disease, autism or facial paralysis, affect a person's emotional expression – as we saw with Kathleen Bogart.

Most theorists, including Barrett, don't address such factors, and nor do they consider what happens as faces age. Ekman's studies used younger faces because they are seen as easier to code. Older faces become less readable, as brows get furrowed, mouths turn down and jowls develop. But emotions also change over our lives, as the Galenic theorists knew – the emotions a young man feels in response to a slight probably won't be the same as those of an elderly woman.

And what of the presumptions we make about older people? How often have they felt misunderstood because of inadvertently seeming to be mean, unkind or irritable? I am often told by my adult children that I look grumpy or bad-tempered when I am nothing of the sort (we are back to the gendered notion of 'resting bitch face'). I can't even blame this on ageing; when I was a teenager, a boy called me 'the girl who always looks like she's about to cry'.

Some of us aren't good at hiding what we are feeling, or reading the faces of others. People with neurodivergence, such as autism, can find the analysis of facial expression bewildering, especially when the words are saying something different. This can sometimes reflect a more evolved, empathic skill of reading – we might notice a cognitive dissonance when there is a mismatch between face and words ('I love you,' he might say, with the eyes of a dead fish).

Those of us with a history of interpersonal trauma might also become hyper-vigilant, attuned to every single flicker of emotion that passes over another person's face. And some introverts worry about what their faces are supposed to be doing in social gatherings – many of us felt like that after the pandemic lockdowns ended, leaving us rusty at the art of conversation.

This all matters because there's a high price to be paid for getting it wrong – not just interpersonally, most of us can cope with that, but in judicial contexts. Judges and juries often interpret facial expressions as evidence of remorse, guilt or sincerity, and harsher sentencing can result if a person doesn't display the 'appropriate' emotions. A 2005 article in the *Canadian Journal of Criminology and Criminal Justice* found that visible evidence of remorse was key to sentencing, but what happens if you don't have a 'sympathetic' enough face – or are innocent? And there are other studies that show the reverse – that if you look guilty (whatever that means), jurors will presume that you are.

Along with the attractiveness of a defendant and their perceived likeability, their emotional expression also influences jury decisions. Look at the American Amanda Knox, who in 2007 was charged with the murder of her flatmate Meredith Kercher in Perugia, Italy. Although the sentence was eventually overturned, she was found guilty in large part because of her demeanour – she was viewed as 'cold' and 'detached' because she didn't show visible emotion, and Italian prosecutors cited her lack of tears as evidence of guilt. It is especially controversial if a woman doesn't show grief; like Lady Macbeth she can be regarded as calculating and contrary to nature.

Racial prejudice comes into play too. Some 40 per cent of all prisoners in the U.S. are Black, as are 50 per cent of those later exonerated; yet they make up only 13 per cent of the American population. In the court room, the 'angry Black man' trope means that even if a man *is* innocent, he is more likely to be treated as guilty, especially if the case involves interpersonal violence. And if we feel more sympathy towards people who look like us, then the lack of diversity on the benches is a problem – only 11 per cent of judges in the U.S. are Black (1.3 per cent in the U.K.).

From Le Brun's standardized emotions to Ekman's universal expressions, we have repeatedly sought simple rules for complex emotions. Like physiognomy, pathognomy is popular because it is easy to use and reproducible. It is also lazy thinking; to reduce an emotion to a single expression and a person to a face benefits the status quo, and those who have something to sell.

The pressing question is not whether we can read emotions in the face – of course we can, sometimes. But what we are reading is not neutral and we often get it wrong. And expressions of emotions are whole-body experiences not just facial ones. Yes, we emote with our face, but we also emote with our posture, gestures, touch, clothes, hair, voice, breath and even our scent.

Every time we look at a person and think we know what they are feeling, we're participating in a practice that is part art, part science, part projection. Until we acknowledge that reading emotions is as much about power as science, and as much about our cultural assumptions as anything else, then we will build the future on the errors of the past.

It is heartening, then, that the tide is turning. In 2020, Microsoft's Azure Face withdrew public access to emotion-recognition software. It was found that the software cannot accurately interpret emotions; it failed to understand meanings from context; and in common with algorithmic biases around beauty, it performed badly with ethnic differences. We saw in the chapter on photography that the algorithms for colour processing are skewed by colour; and in Azure Face, people with darker skin tones often had their emotions represented incorrectly.

The story of facial expression is ultimately a story about power – who gets to define what the face is saying, whose expression is considered normal or abnormal, whose face is read as trustworthy or dangerous. Whether it is Kathleen Bogart's doctor making a presumption about her intelligence based on her face, or a facial-recognition system announcing we are a terrorist, these judgements are all too often based on the same flawed assumptions that have surrounded the face for centuries.

So, what do we do about this? Plenty – in terms of building holistic systems, changing the way we use training data, reframing the problems, and pushing for regulatory frameworks.

It is clear that technology is never neutral – from photography to facial-recognition systems – and that messy history should be part of how we build AI systems. Historians and anthropologists are less favoured by developers than psychologists; we have an 'it's complicated' approach to cultural meaning, which is harder to use as a hook than 'there are six emotions; happiness looks like this and sadness like this.' But don't we deserve systems that reflect our human complexity – and are at least freer from bias?

The legacy of Victorian science on the ways we look at the world, and how we categorize, measure and think about humanity, is so pervasive that we barely notice it. It is there in our intellectual frameworks, our language, our academic disciplines and medical systems, as well as our civic institutions.

In national museums and galleries, which were so important to the Victorians in making a public statement about human and social progress, archaeologists and anthropologists have feverishly worked – and continue to work – on the creation of three-dimensional faces. We use the face as a storytelling device, whether the stories are about empire, or industry, or evolution.

We find the same drive in other reconstructions of the face – whether it's Madame Tussaud making death masks of guillotined aristocrats, or modern forensic teams reconstructing famous faces from Tutankhamun to Shakespeare. We want to know what people 'really' looked like.

Why? For the same reason that we care about emotional expression, and that we carry about the image of a loved one; and for the same reason that we want our own faces captured for posterity. Because faces are the clue to our social identity and emotional connection – at an individual and a social level; right or wrong, we believe that we know a person better, that we understand who they are, once we have gazed into their eyes.

But what if the face is a fiction? What if it contains more art than science? What if it tells us more about ourselves than anyone else? Does any of that matter? Let's turn to the science of forensic facial reconstruction and find out.

7.
Reconstructed

Since 2014 a bust of Richard III has occupied a plinth at a Visitor Centre named after him in Leicester (fig. 28). The model is based on a CT scan of the king's skull, and printed in plastic, using a technique called stereolithography. It depicts Richard before his defeat by Henry Tudor at the Battle of Bosworth in 1485, a battle that ended the Plantagenet dynasty. Nearly five and a half centuries later, Richard's face, fixed for ever at thirty-three years old, is mottled pink, with thick eyebrows, dark hair and a half smile. On his head sits a black hat with a glamorous pin, a replica brass filigree set with a ruby red stone, four hematite octagon stones and four pearls – based on the one shown in his most famous (sixteenth-century) portrait.

This is a kindlier, more contemplative face than you might expect to see on a man vilified by William Shakespeare as a 'villain' inside and out, a prince-murdering coward with a hunch back, a withered arm and a limp.

In 2024 the face of Shanidar Z, a 75,000-year-old Neanderthal woman, was similarly reconstructed from human remains; with the aid of digital scanning and 3D printing, 200 bone fragments were assembled from a 'flat as a pancake' skull found in a cave in Iraqi Kurdistan (fig. 29). Nothing is known about Shanidar Z; her name is an invention – Shanidar is the name of the cave in which the skull was found. The model wears no clothes, and has long dark hair that covers her shoulders. She has a weathered and dark complexion, and ambiguous ethnicity; her brow is lifted to form a quizzical expression and her mouth seems kindly and patient.

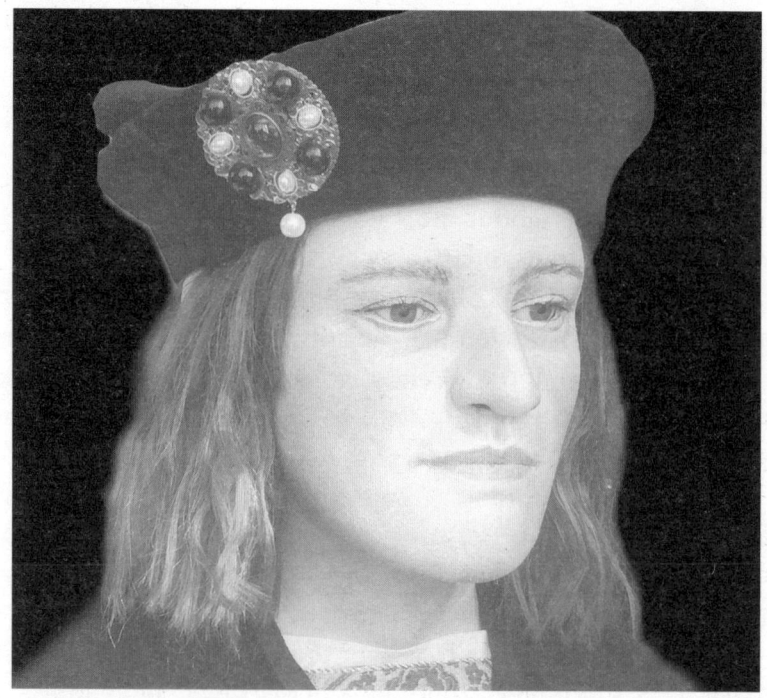

28. Caroline Wilkinson, Reconstruction of Richard III, 2012.

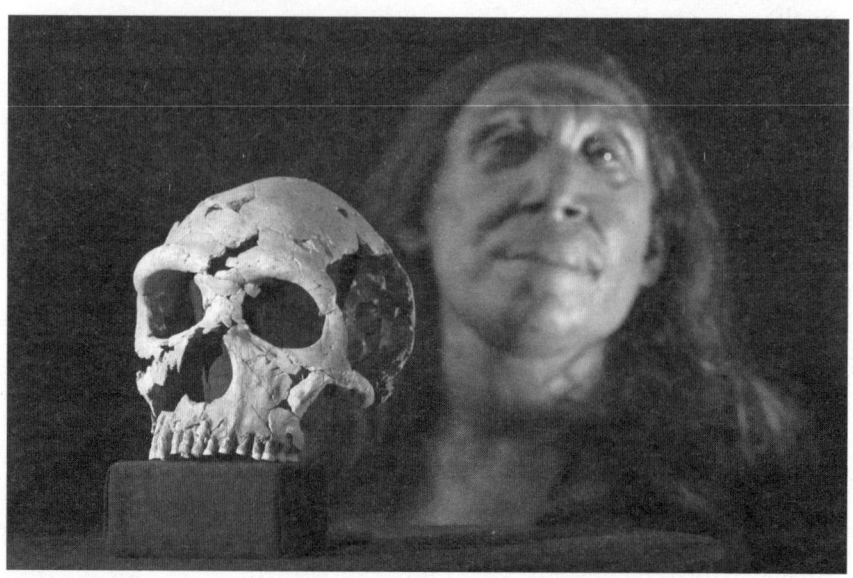

29. Adrie and Alfons Kennis, the face of Shanidar Z, 2024.

At first glance, these historical reconstructions have little in common – one is a monarch who since his death has been memorialized in history, portraits and plays; the other an unknown woman, buried with a rock for a pillow. But in both instances, the careful reconstruction of the face contributes to detailed, powerful and emotive testimony about the identity of a person, and what their existence means to us today.

Both Richard III and Shanidar Z are presented as scientific renderings, offering a version of a person that is intended to be more real, authentic-looking and emotionally engaging than a 2D image. In both, this is achieved through the facial expression, skin tone and direction of the eye gaze; they put 'a face to a name', even if Shanidar Z's name is an invention.

Picture yourself as an artist staring at a bare skull, trying to imagine the living person who once inhabited it. How might you go about reconstructing that face?

It's a different question than a surgeon would confront, but there are parallels; this is an aesthetic as well as a practical task, and many artists have spent years training in anatomical dissection – they are well versed in how a face fits on a skull.

When there is no soft tissue to work with, a forensic artist will examine the skull and recreate a 3D rendering. Specific landmarks, features on the bone's surface, are overlayed with clay that approximates tissue depth. The earliest studies measured that information from cadavers, but now modern ultrasound and CT scanning technologies are used to collect comparative data from the living. Before the clay is applied to the skull, researchers consider the profile of the jawbones, the symmetry and size of the nasal bones, the state of the teeth.

Forensic artist Joe Mullins, senior forensic imaging specialist at the National Center for Missing and Exploited Children in the U.S., describes the process as 'doing a portrait, but we're doing it from the inside out'. The skull is the armature, the framework on which everything is constructed. 'Doesn't matter if you're male or female, Black, white, Asian,' Joe told me. 'The muscles leave marks on the skull. So that gives us a good baseline.'

Joe will collaborate with anthropologists, who use physical facts about the skeleton to determine a person's years, gender and origins. He can then use the average tissue depths for people of the appropriate age, sex and ethnicity. The information on muscularity and the tissue-depth markers allows him to outline the contours of the face onto the shape of the skull, thus giving a fair representation of how the eyelids, eyebrows, hairline, ears, nose and lips would have sat.

'It's not just making a face,' Joe tells me. 'It's sculpting the right face to go with that skull.'

On YouTube you can see videos of Joe at work – he marks with safety matches areas that are attached to a cast of a skull; those markers correspond to the calculations of soft tissue, fat pads, the position of the eyes, the brows, the chin. Then he moulds the features from clay. On one occasion Joe worked with sculpture students from the New York Academy of Art to recreate the faces of eleven unidentified crime victims.

Joe's motivation might be different from paleo-artists', who bring ancient people to life. But the skills used to reconstruct Shanidar Z or Richard III, or a missing person, originated in the nineteenth century. Today those skills are added to by CT scanning and 3D printing – which the artist Caroline Wilkinson used to model Richard III's skin and muscles, along with portraits to get the skin tone, hair and eye colour right.

But here's something that might surprise you: people in earlier periods did fashion faces from skulls, long before the tools we use today. Neolithic people, from 9,000–7,000 years ago, buried skulls separately from bodies; some were found in Jericho, covered in clay with cowrie shells in the eye sockets.

That act alone, of keeping and decorating the head, suggests that the body might have had a lesser role in ideas of the person, long before facehood as we know it. Skin tone and facial features were painted onto the surface of the dried plaster, presumably invoking the look of the person who had lived.

We don't know the purpose of these skulls, though anthropologists think they were symbolic and representative, rather than a pursuit of likeness – which is in keeping with what we have learned in this book about portraiture.

This drive to see faces from the past connects us directly to our ancestors, but it also reveals how our understanding of human identity has evolved. The earliest modern attempts at historical reconstruction were developed in the late 1800s by the German anatomist Hermann Welcker and the Swiss anatomist Wilhelm His, Sr, working in two areas that were later central to anthropology: the study of human differences and archaeology.

Welcker and His collaborated with artists to visualize Neanderthals, and other early hominids, and to describe human evolution; they based their findings on evidence drawn from other sciences, such as craniometry, as used by the French physician Paul Broca (whom we will meet again in chapter eight), and the Swedish anatomist Anders Retzius.

You will not be surprised, given all we have learned about Victorian categorization, that they predicted intelligence and ethnicity by reading skulls, which tied people into the racial hierarchies underpinning scientific racism. Some attempt was made in early historical reconstruction to be precise, but they mostly conformed to racial presumptions – especially after the 'Old Man of La Chapelle' was discovered, in 1908, in a cave in La Chapelle-aux-Saints in south-central France (fig. 30). Based on this find, the first relatively complete skeleton of its kind, and on the previous century of anthropological research, Edwardian scientists created images of Neanderthals that were reproduced around the Western world. Imagine walking through the Museum of Natural History in Paris in the early 1900s and encountering these striking reconstructions. The palaeontologist Marcellin Boule and the artist Charles R. Knight depicted simian and ape-like models, with Neanderthals hunched and dumblooking in comparison to modern humans.

It was a story of human progress. Similar models appeared in the U.S. and the U.K. where Neanderthal families with stooped postures and apelike features scavenged and lived in harsh conditions. These were failures, by the standards of the 1930s consumers we met in

The Face

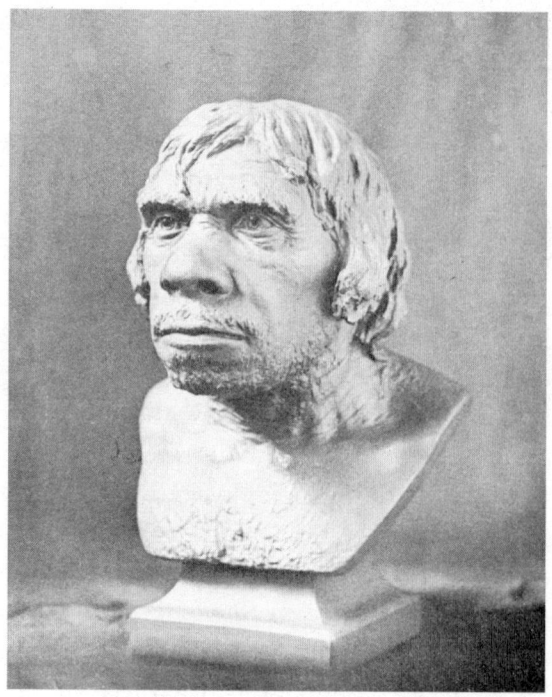

30. Unknown artist, *The Old Man of La Chapelle-aux-Saints*, 1908.

our chapter on mirrors, and delberately different from those who, in just a few decades, would land on the moon.

The interested public who devoured accounts of ancient Egyptian tombs, prehistoric cave art and prehistoric remains wanted to know what people from the past looked like. Remember how important photography had been for the Victorians, for whom seeing was believing? These exercises in historical reconstruction gave Victorians and Edwardians alike a sense of scientific mastery over their past: history was made visible and tangible, just for them, no matter that it was based on little actual evidence.

Consider the case of 'Java Man' or *Pithecanthropus erectus*, now classified as *Homo erectus*, which the Dutch paleoanthropologist Eugène Dubois found in Indonesia in 1891. This was pitched as the missing link between apes and humans, but the fossilized remains recovered were sparse – a tooth, a partial skullcap or cranium, and a femur, or thigh bone. The skullcap had a low, elongated profile, with a prominent brow ridge and thick bone walls, traits that were associated with primitive hominids and apes. But the brain size was estimated to be transitional from humans to apes. The tooth also had similar features to modern humans, as did the femur; the combination of a human-like femur with a primitive skullcap was enough to convince Dubois that *Pithecanthropus erectus* was an upright-walking ape-man.

Later finds, including more complete fossils, showed that *Homo erectus* was closer to modern humans than to apes, but in Dubois' time his interpretation supported the 'ape-like' ancestry of certain people. As private collections were turned into public museums that made statements about the Western world and its imperial past, skulls from indigenous people, collected by ethnographers, were used to reconstruct faces.

In the dioramas at museums such as the Pitt Rivers in Oxford, the relationship between skull and face shape was a well-established focus of evolutionary studies. Once again, the story was teleological, meaning that it progressed from the primitive to the civilized. The Smithsonian's Natural History Museum's 'Africa' exhibit took the visitor from Black 'savagery' to white enlightenment.

As a child I was taken to the Pitt Rivers and lifted up to look in the glass cases filled with shrunken heads; I was transfixed. Today there is much more awareness of the ethical problems in displaying human remains and many museums have removed their dioramas from display. Some national museums, including the British Museum, continue to display human remains, most famously Egyptian mummies, but others have them in storage, carefully tended and preserved and argued over.

The transformation of facial reconstruction from these troubling beginnings into a more sophisticated science began in earnest during the twentieth century. Then, facial reconstruction underwent a significant transformation as scientific advancements in forensic anthropology influenced historical reconstructions. The development of methods such as tissue depth markers helped show the plumpness of a cheek or the boniness of a jawline, and the Soviet archaeologist and anthropologist Mikhail Gerasimov applied these techniques not only to criminal investigations but also to the faces of historical figures, bridging the gap between forensic science and historical inquiry.

Gerasimov studied the skulls and reconstructed the faces of more than 200 people, ranging from the earliest excavated *Homo sapiens* and Neanderthals to medieval monarchs and dignitaries. He wrote about these cases in his 1968 autobiography *The Face Finder*, as opportunities to 'gaze on the faces of those long dead'. The term 'face finder' implies that the face is waiting there to be discovered – though it is also imagined and brought into being.

By the 1970s, tissue markers were supported by CT scanning that provided more detailed examination of craniofacial anatomy. In addition to research on cadavers that were approximated for gender, race and age, these new techniques gave facial reconstruction a legitimacy that allowed it to cross over from bioarchaeology into criminal investigations of missing persons undertaken by artists such as Joe Mullins.

Think about what this work means beyond the science. Facial reconstruction can be a moral mission as well as an artistic one; it returns identity to people whose bodies were found in dumpsters and side streets, murdered and abandoned. Carmen Bilton, one of Joe Mullins's students, described why this process mattered so much to her, as a human being as well as an artist: 'I want to get it right so that somebody can recognise her. Because she was somebody. She was a real person.'

Without a face, personhood is lost. The same sentiment is expressed by plastic and reconstructive surgeons who seek to repair faces damaged by accidents, violence, fires or disease.

You might think, watching television shows, that forensic reconstruction captures the attention of the public in missing-person reports, just as it does in museums. But the practice is not as commonplace as people think. In popular American television series such as *Bones*, which unite the FBI with forensic anthropologists and forensic archaeologists, a reconstructed face is produced the moment skeletal remains are found. Angela Montenegro, the fictional forensic reconstruction specialist in *Bones*, uses 3D technology and holograms to 'give victims back their faces'.

But this work is rare outside of fiction. It is time-consuming and requires considerable skill. This is why thousands of unidentified skulls line the vaults of American police stations, their identity listed only as cold cases. Why aren't these skulls being reconstructed?

Part of the answer is financial – a lack of investment. And we don't know for certain how successful it is. If a person is identified because of the reconstruction, artists won't necessarily get the credit for it, or even be told; there's no incentive for busy police forces to feed back on the outcomes. Another reason is training – there are only so many Joe Mullins in the world.

Moreover, not enough people care; without names, people are invisible; naming closes the loop on the face, the person and their identity. It is akin to the engagement trick used in charity marketing, where there is usually a specific, named child asking for help, her small face and wide eyes appealing to you as a fellow human. A single person's death is a tragedy, a thousand deaths is a statistic, as the saying goes; we need the particularity of personhood to feel empathy, and unidentified corpses have – well – no identity.

And yet, some faces matter more than ever before, as we have seen throughout this book, and there are new digital technologies available to give faces to the long dead. A mummified Peruvian girl who was ritually sacrificed 500 years ago was discovered in 1995; thirty years later she was given a fresh face and a new name: Juanita. The 8,300-year-old remains of a young boy found in a cave in Norway in 1917 became the 'Boy from Viste', evoked as 'The Lonely Ice-Age Boy'. His face was reconstructed in 2023, so he now has a face, an emotional state, and a name that aligns with the twenty-first-century 'loneliness pandemic'.

Such historical examples are reported as scientific breakthroughs – but how much are they about science? Just one example provides a clue about the complex interplay between scientific method and human assumption: the case of the Vasa ship, which set sail from

Stockholm harbour on its maiden voyage on 10 August 1628. She had barely sailed 1,300 metres before she sank – a structural deficiency meant that in light wind she capsized and toppled, taking fifty-three lives with her. The ship remained underwater until 1961, when she was brought to the surface – along with eighteen skeletons.

The Vasa ship got her own museum in 1990, but it wasn't until 2006 that historical reconstructions were sought. The Swedish artist Oscar Nilsson was commissioned by the Vasa Museum to make faces for six of the eighteen skeletons, one of whom was nicknamed Gustav. Osteologists, bone specialists, recorded that the skeleton belonged to a man in his mid-forties, and that he was the shortest man on board. Hard work had caused problems with his back, and the skull looked masculine, the artist recalled, 'with a squarish facial shape and rather heavy jaw and chin'. Using that information, Nilsson made a model of Gustav: 'I was very pleased with the result: a man of hard work, with beard stubble and hair on his chest. But . . . there was a big surprise coming up, years later.'

That surprise came in the form of DNA testing. DNA can reveal whether a skeleton is male or female by analysing genetic markers on the sex chromosomes; biologically female skeletons typically have XX chromosomes and biologically male skeletons typically XY ones. Tests on Gustav revealed that she was in fact female; twenty-five to thirty years old, not forty-five, and blonde. Even though there were women on board, it had apparently not occurred to any of the scientists involved, in 2006, that Gustav might be female.

Such gendered ideas aren't new – the historian Londa Schiebinger showed how eighteenth-century scientists identified the sex of a skeleton by assuming women had smaller skulls and larger pelvises: they saw what they wanted to see. Today we recognize that individuals vary; female pelvises aren't always larger than men's and their skulls aren't always smaller. But we still see what we expect to see – in 2017, DNA evidence found that the skeleton of a Viking warrior presumed to be male had XX chromosomes. The grave was filled with weapons, and it didn't occur to anybody that the warrior could have been female. Such discoveries upend historical clichés and certainties.

Reconstructed

And what did it mean for Gustav? Well, Nilsson had to start again with his reconstruction, 'rebuilding the face from the skull but this time with female measurements', making some alterations to reflect her age, and with new knowledge about the colours of her eyes, her skin and her hair. In deciding what colours to make Gertrude's face, skin and eyes, Nilsson relied on the categories used by geneticists. DNA indicates hair and eye colour; it's considered 80 per cent accurate, and for skin tones in DNA analysis there are five established groups: very pale, pale, medium, dark and very dark. To create Gertrude's feminine features, Nilsson used modern Scandinavian and Northern European statistics about physical appearance from women who were roughly the same age.

And just like that, Gustav became Gertrude, a blonde, blue-eyed Scandinavian woman (fig. 31 and 32). The only distinctive aspect of her appearance is larger than usual ears, based on prominent mastoids – bones found just behind the ears. Joe Mullins does not give his reconstructed faces skin or hair colour; in case it is incorrect and

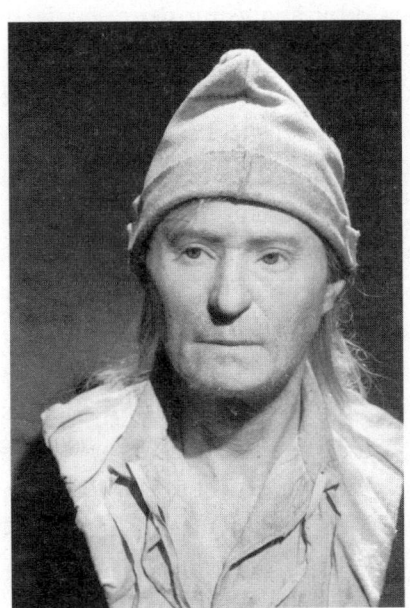

31. Oscar Nilsson, *Gustav* (2006).

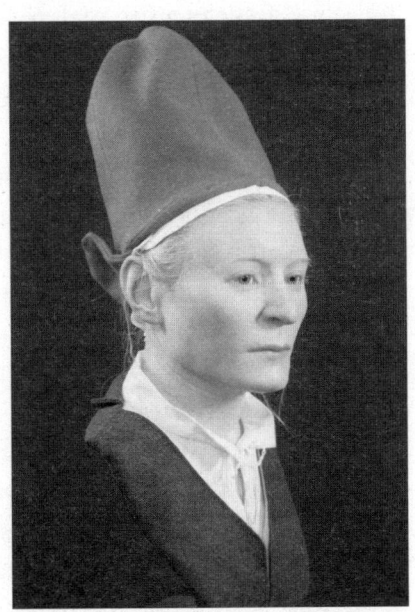

32. Oscar Nilsson, *Gertrude* (2023).

hinders identification. But Gertrude's face and eyes are coloured, so that visitors to the Vasa Museum see more in her to relate to – rather as Victorian photographs of street urchins are colourized and shared on Facebook; somehow adding colour makes people feel 'more like us'.

Gertrude became, with these subtle changes, someone familiar. Her physicality, her weight, was guesswork, as there is no tissue-depth analysis from the seventeenth century. As we have seen, the earliest ones date from the late nineteenth century. Nilsson made her thin, because in the seventeenth century people lived more hand-to-mouth than they do today. Osteologists and forensic geneticists can also advise artists in this area, as dental condition can indicate malnourishment.

As far as he could, Nilsson relied on the scientific evidence that was available to him, but clearly what he saw in the skull when he thought it was male, was different from what he saw when he knew it was female. This led to a series of artistic choices. At some point, he says, after the face has been covered with an initial layer of clay for the skin, 'I need to use my artistic skills to make the face come alive'.

The science might provide the basis of a face, but it is art that gives the face character and identity: 'I try to add as subtle and soft expressions as I can to create the impression of a real human face. It can be just enough with letting the eyes look to the side, or a turning of the head. I try to be very aware of not describing a personality, but to give the impression that there is a consciousness behind the eyes, life. I am aware that my reconstructions are a bit too beautiful: it is most speculative to add stuff like skin problems or oddly shaped ears.'

We can see the artistry involved when we compare the faces of Gustav and Gertrude, both of which remain on display at the Vasa Museum, accompanied by the story of their change. The feminization of Gertrude is apparent in her skin tone and texture and her larger lips, all of which are based on modern images of women who are younger than Gustav was. Gertrude's nose points down less than Gustav's did, which Nilsson attributes to new DNA evidence. But it also provides a more feminine appearance. She appears much less harassed and tired than Gustav – a reflection of her younger age, or a reference to modern ideas about feminine attractiveness?

Nilsson wanted to 'show a woman marked by strenuous work but with an awareness of the tragic event that marked her end'. We don't know what work Gertrude would have been doing on the ship; women are now known to have been on warships more often than previously thought – not as sailors or warriors, but as sex workers, or wives, since they were allowed to accompany their husbands in home waters. But what of her back, strained by repeated heavy lifting?

As to what 'Gertrude is thinking about', Nilsson adds, 'I leave that to all visitors to the museum.' But the interpretation is also given by the artist; we do not know whether Gertrude was aware of her end; we know nothing about her life or her experience of being on the ship. Nor do we know whether she was wearing a fashionable red hat; Nilsson added that touch because one was found nearby.

When we recreate a face, we necessarily create stories and mythologies around them – sometimes they are individual, and sometimes national, as we see with Richard III. The king's remains were retrieved in 2012 from beneath a car park in Leicester. He had lain in that spot since his ignominious defeat at Bosworth on 22 August 1485. The drama around retrieval of the bones was made into at least two actual dramas – one for BBC television and the other as a cinematic release, starring the comedian and writer Steve Coogan. In both, the discovery of Richard's remains was depicted as the culmination of a sole and dogged crusade by Philippa Langley, Secretary of the Richard III Society. Again, we like to put a face to an idea – in this case, Philippa's.

Richard III has not been a beloved king in the popular imagination. He is still best known as the likely murderer of the 'Princes in the Tower', his two nephews, the rightful heirs to the throne after Richard deposed another nephew, Edward V. Did Richard kill his nephews to make himself king? And did he also kill his wife – another claim – who was too old to bear him an heir? We will never know, but images of King Richard were deliberately altered to suggest that this was the kind of man who might have.

At least two dozen portraits were made of Richard III, most of them posthumously. In decorating the great houses of Elizabethan England, as we saw in our chapter on portraiture, it was common to commission portraits. Rich people often showed off sets that stretched back as far as William the Conqueror, hoping to convey an idea of the family's own grandeur and ancient lineage. Many portraits of Richard III are based on one held by the British Royal Collections, in which the king wears black velvet and gold brocade, with that famous hat and brooch. He is placing a ring on the little finger of his right hand, typically a symbol of union (fig. 33).

As a portrait, this painting is intended to resemble the king, rather than to suggest any psychological interiority. Contemporaries, and

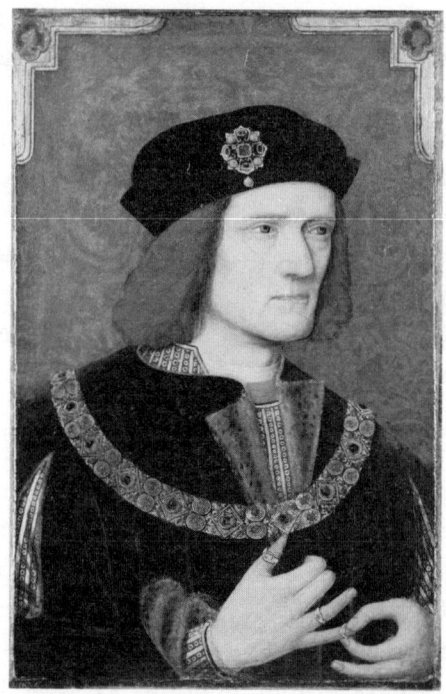

33. Unknown artist, *Richard III*, early 16th century portrait.

later critics like Shakespeare, used the portrait as evidence of the king's cruel nature – his expression and features have been described as cold and calculating, and there are echoes of physiognomic convention in his small eyes and narrow lips. So how far was the image a likeness? It is hard to know. Little was recorded about him while he was living, and accounts produced after his death were not flattering.

According to the scholar Sir Thomas More, Henry VIII's unfortunate Chancellor, Richard was a short man, with a crooked back, uneven shoulders and a mean-looking face: 'hard-favoured of visage . . . malicious, wrathful, envious'. More was only eight when Richard died at the Battle of Bosworth, but this description has stuck. Shakespeare used and perpetuated it in his personification of Richard as a 'bottled spider' and a 'poisonous bunch-back'd toad'.

But here's where the story gets interesting: this painting has been altered since its original composition in around 1510. Art historians have used X-ray technologies to show that in addition to the shoulders being altered to give an imbalance, his eyes and lips were thinned out to give that mean expression. The resulting image is consistent with Polydore Vergil's description in his *Anglica Historia*, commissioned by Richard's usurper Henry VII, in which Richard 'has a short face with an expression that was harsh and cruel'. Was the painting adjusted to fit the propaganda of the Tudor court, to depict Richard III as physically and morally weak and corrupt? Probably. If Richard was a villain, Henry VII's claim to the throne would be stronger.

Since the discovery of Richard III's skeleton, there has been a drive to rehabilitate him, which is where the reconstructed face comes in. Caroline Wilkinson used modern technologies of reconstruction and anatomical analyses of the skull; she made the lips and the eyes larger, which somewhat undoes the propaganda of the portrait. And when new evidence came in, Caroline made some subtle enhancements; DNA testing revealed that the king's hair would have been lighter and his eyes blue, so the brown eyes were swapped, and a new wig added. She tells me that another wig is being made, to reflect new findings made about his hairstyle.

Giving Richard III a friendlier face no doubt improves his public

The Face

reputation – as does placing that face within a Visitor Centre dedicated to information about the reign of an 'anointed king of England'. At the Centre, the visitor follows a detective story to find out how Richard III's skeleton was found in the car park, magically beneath the letter R – for reserved, but mysteriously also for Rex; how the site was once home to Greyfriars Church, which was dissolved during Henry VIII's destruction of the monasteries, when the land passed into private hands – and eventually to Leicester City Council. A replica skeleton can be viewed in the Visitor Centre, where you can also stand over and gaze at the grave where the skeleton was found.

There is a mystical, fairy-tale quality to this story of the king's rediscovery and reinterment; his actual remains were interred at Leicester Cathedral, in a ceremony presided over by the Archbishop of Canterbury, and with a reading by the actor Benedict Cumberbatch, who is a distant relative of Richard III (rather than merely sharing some very distant ancestor – which would be the case for most Europeans).

What happens when one comes 'face to face' with the reconstructed Richard III? For the independent historian John Ashdown-Hill, who wrote several books about Richard III and collaborated with Philippa Langley, it was an emotional experience. 'I previously said when I stood by the grave in Leicester that I felt closer to Richard III than I had ever been, but when I saw the facial reconstruction, I felt almost in the presence of a living Richard III.'

Philippa was even more explicit about the emotional pull of the face, and the impact made by a favourable reconstruction: 'It doesn't look like the face of a tyrant. I'm sorry but it doesn't. He's very handsome. It's like you could just talk to him, have a conversation with him right now.'

Of course, tyrants can be handsome, but what matters is that both John and Philippa were reacting emotionally to the proximity of a reconstructed face – that is, to the basic human intimacy of looking into the eyes of another. But there is more to it than that. I have stood in front of that historical reconstruction and felt no emotional connection – but Richard III does not have the same significance for me that he does for John and Philippa.

Not all faces provoke a human connection then. What we feel when we look at another person's face depends on our relationship, our cultural beliefs, the artistry involved and the meanings we give to that face. For example, alongside any emotional response or sense of kinship we see in a fellow human, a reconstructed king might spark a surge of the kind of loyalty that anchors 'us' in a shared national history.

So, what happens when we construct a Neanderthal? It might provoke us to feel that we are looking at something related to us but different from us – which takes us back to the Victorians, and those dioramas of human origins.

From archaeological findings, we know that Neanderthals had quite different faces to you and me. They were larger with bigger foreheads and protruding noses; some researchers have related the latter to evolutionary adaptation – prominent noses can help moisten and regulate air that is breathed in. This was useful in the hotter climate of the Middle East, before Neanderthals migrated to cooler regions of Europe, adapting to longer winters and low-light environments. Neanderthals also had slightly larger brains than modern humans, with wider faces and jaws without the bony chin we have. Their teeth and jaws were designed for chewing raw meat and leveraging as tools.

Our projecting chins might reflect dietary changes – our jaws became smaller as our ancestors started tenderizing meat by cooking it with fire. It is possible that the chin might have evolved for social reasons; more nuanced emotional communication would have developed as human societies grew larger and more complex. Could the chin have helped convey feelings? We don't know – certainly, today, people can have Botox to correct an over-expressive chin that 'cobbles', creating a peach-pit effect.

Neanderthals also had bigger eye sockets than we do – some evolutionary biologists suggest this meant better vision, especially in low-light environments such as long winters in Europe and parts of

Asia. But as we have learned from other organs, bigger isn't always better. Larger eye sockets might have meant that more of Neanderthals' brainpower was devoted to visual processing, leaving less left-brain activity for cognitive functions like social interaction.

This remaking of the human face is one of the most neglected, and most critical, aspects of studying evolutionary development. Most research into the evolutionary development of Neanderthals focuses on the brain rather than the face, largely because skulls survive and give clues to brain size and shape, whereas faces do not. That is why early historical reconstructions clutched at what scientists believed they did know – they gave Neanderthals a low, receding forehead, protruding midface and heavy brow; the same baseness and stupidity they thought they found among 'lower races'.

Scientists saw in skulls, and faces, what they saw or wanted to see, to explain how we ended up with modern humans. They saw 'progress' and the dying out of those who didn't measure up as evidence of the 'survival of the fittest' – an expression erroneously attributed to Darwin (instead of the social philosopher Herbert Spencer). And they saw evidence of the superiority of white people over those whom they cast as being, or resembling, colonial subjects and slaves.

Once such visual images have been locked into the popular imagination, they are difficult to dislodge. It is an example of the 'anchor bias' we discussed in our chapter on perfecting the face. Who knows what kinds of scientific development may have been stunted or derailed as a result?

For decades the Neanderthals described in the early 1900s, along with those dioramas of Victorian evolution that progressed from apes to savages, set the scene for understanding human evolution. The white, Western imperialist guardians of civilization decreed that these were not 'people like us', so they didn't bother to give them emotions, or indeed any meaningful connection with modern humans.

Today, we see Neanderthals differently, and this is reflected in their faces. The historical reconstruction of Shanidar Z, based on research at Cambridge University, invites us to empathize and see her story, the story of Neanderthals, as part of human history. 'I think she can help us connect with who [Neanderthals] were,' said paleo-archaeologist Emma Pomeroy, a member of the research team on a new Netflix/BBC documentary, *Secrets of the Neanderthals*.

Pomeroy described the reconstruction of Shanidar Z's skull as a 'high-stakes 3D jigsaw puzzle'. Researchers took micro-CT scans of the fossilized bones and pieced together the skull before it was scanned, then 3D printed. That formed the basis of the head made by the Dutch paleo-artist twin brothers Adrie and Alfons Kennis, who built up layers of fabricated muscle and skin to produce the face we see today.

Along with John Gurche, best known for his beautiful renderings at the Smithsonian, the Kennis brothers are responsible for some of the most celebrated facial reconstructions in the world – including at the Natural History Museum in London. The Museum's website announces the models in the Human Evolution gallery to be 'two of the most scientifically accurate reconstructions that exist'. Visitors can stare 'into the twinkling eyes in the weathered features of the Neanderthal man' and 'feel a moment of connection, of recognising another fellow human, albeit of a different species'. Again, we see that invocation to 'connection' as an emotional and instinctive sense, rather than a factual one.

Once the facial muscles have been laid down according to scientific measurements, a face might start to look like a face, but it's not yet characterful or engaging – these qualities come through in movement and expression, and creating the sense of a person being a person requires considerable artistic skill. It is noticeable especially around the eyes and to a lesser degree the mouth, artists tell me – which is the same thing I have been told by plastic surgeons and robotic engineers. This is because our gaze is drawn first to eyes, and then to mouths – the places that are most important in human communication: Can you see me? Will you speak to me?

As for the shape and 'fullness of the lips, the shape of the nostrils, the shape of the tip of the nose, the folds of the eyes', Alfons Kennis says that these are created according to the judgement and skills of the artist. Caroline Wilkinson disagrees – at least when it comes to the thickness of the lips, which tend to follow the line of the teeth; big teeth equate to big lips, on average. What teeth can't indicate is the shape of the lips, and whether the person had that feature of the upper lip known as the Cupid's bow.

These differences between the perspectives of artists are important, for there is as much art as science in Shanidar Z's face. Most portrait sculptors working from life will start by measuring the distances and angles of their model's head with callipers and a notebook; for the dead, technologies such as DNA testing, 3D scans and CT imaging offer the artist the scaffolding on which to overlay identity. When an artist creates a face from the past, they can't avoid drawing on present-day presumptions, and their own cognitive bias – shaped by personal feelings, beliefs, environment, training and even mood.

All faces are products of culture and environment as much as skeletal structure – as each of the chapters in this book show. It is true that we can know from the shape of the bones and brow if an individual had a pronounced forehead or other baseline facial structures. But even if we can work out how the person's facial muscles, nerves and fibres overlaid the skull, there's a limit to the scientific evidence available.

The elements that bring a sculpture or artwork to life, and perhaps elevate it to being more than a portrait, are the subtle details: the ways in which skin colour and texture are imagined, the suggestion of forehead lines or the hint of a half-smile. It's in the twinkle of an eye or the crinkle of a cheek – those fleeting qualities that truly create a sense of connection, that can make us like or dislike or fall in love with a person.

So, what do we do to Neanderthal faces when we overlay skeletal remains with such modern affects? We are bringing them back into the fold, asserting that they are 'just like us' and not club-wielding thugs, which is how the Old Man of La Chapelle was imagined. And we do this for a very specific but unacknowledged reason.

Neanderthals were once thought to be a separate species to modern humans; now it is recognized that we interbred.

Modern humans share around 99 per cent of their DNA with chimpanzees and a little more with Neanderthals. We share an evolutionary history with both species, and Neanderthals left a small but lasting imprint on the human gene pool. This awareness confirmed anthropologists' belief that Neanderthals were less brutish and savage than we once thought; offering as evidence the facts that Neanderthals had burial practices, cared for the sick and created what seems to be art.

Clearly the recognition of a shared DNA moves the narrative of human evolution away from the notion of *Homo sapiens* as modern successors who outwitted Neanderthals. Perhaps it also reframes the process of evolution as one of collaboration and progress rather than of violence, competition and conquest – though I am always suspicious of 'interbreeding' being cited as cooperation. It goes without saying that pregnancy can be forced.

These are the reasons why Shanidar Z is a world away in appearance from the Old Man of La Chapelle. She looks like a thoughtful, approachable, even kindly middle-aged woman – though since half her teeth were rotten, she might as easily have been tormented, angry and in pain. We do not know whether she would have – or could have – smiled. We have no idea what faces meant to Neanderthals – though, if you remember our discussion of cave paintings, faces weren't commemorated in ways that have survived.

So we cannot know from a skull whether Shanidar Z would have smiled, or expressed emotions in ways that would have created the distinct creases and wrinkles the artists have given her. It has even been debated whether Neanderthals had the same vocal range or hearing as modern humans, which would also have influenced how they communicated emotionally, along with the kinds of relationships they had. Modern humans have complex emotional expressions because they have evolved in complex social groupings – would Neanderthal societies have needed those, or been capable of them?

The beauty of the art behind Shanidar Z is not in question. But we are revealing more about ourselves and our relationship with our early human past and our own faces than about the Neanderthal – we are giving her the things that matter to our sense of modern facehood: a unique facial identity, emotional complexity and a name.

The problem is that we do this without acknowledging that it's what we are doing, and revealing the art behind the science. This means that we don't admit, either, the prejudice that was historically involved in the image of the Neanderthal, or the false versions that made their way into national museums and histories.

Why does this matter? Well, as we have seen throughout this book, there is a long and problematic history of ascribing emotions, intelligence, civility and value to some faces and not to others. Historically, societies have made the faces of those they want to be connected to emotionally empathetic. When cultures have determined that certain groups don't deserve empathy and human compassion, their faces have been subjected to grotesque and inhuman ideas and depictions: anti-Black caricatures from the Jim Crow era and Nazi cartoons of Jewish people are cases in point.

Making faces is one of the most concrete ways in which we can imagine the past. Our fascination today with facial reconstruction of all kinds must relate to the flourishing of popular history in the digital age, and our interest in famous individuals. More television shows and films and documentaries than ever before focus on historical figures, from Elizabeth I to Napoleon, as well as more explicitly fictionalized accounts in novels, plays, children's programmes.

Since the 1980s, Public History has expanded around the world, with academic programmes and organizations being created, and degree and graduate programmes established. And in the age of social media, putting a face to a name matters more than ever before. These two factors probably lie behind the excavation of Richard III's skeleton. After all, people had tried to do it before; at least two campaigners had previously identified where his remains were buried; they just couldn't raise the necessary funds.

The historian Mary Beard has been scathing both about the intellectual value of the discovery and subsequent attempts by the University of Leicester, which takes credit for the discovery, to 'oversell' it. This seems to be a clear case of popular interest trumping academic importance – and what could be more popular than a detective story that involves royal celebrity, murder and Shakespearean intrigue? The excavation made history exciting to an audience that generation after generation has been taught about the Tudors and the Princes in the Tower. In my school we had to read the evidence and determine whether Richard III was guilty. Would our minds have been swayed by Caroline Wilkinson's model and a visit to the Richard III Visitor Centre? Undoubtedly.

Today, we exist in an era of 'historical personages', where famous faces matter most. I have wondered, as I have watched tourists queue outside Madame Tussaud's in London to gaze at the waxwork bodies of the Windsors or Amy Winehouse, whether this is a modern-day kind of pilgrimage, in which the representation matters as much emotionally as the original object itself – the same reason people might buy tea towels emblazoned with the *Mona Lisa*, or postcards, or little prayer cards with pictures of saints on them.

But one thing is clear – even if visitors get a kick out of coming face to face with Richard III, we cannot say whether a king is a killer based on a reconstruction of his face; nor can we claim that a Neanderthal had modern human emotions.

Yes, the face connects us sensorially and emotionally to others, and defines a person's identity, and therefore some faces will always matter more than others. To return to the question I posed earlier: why are we often more concerned with the faces of those we do not know, and can never know, than the faces of missing people?

Often, when a shared nationalistic concept – like monarchical rule – is discussed, the personal provides a way in. There's a reason why magazines have a face on the cover; why journalists like to interview – and photograph – an individual who has been through something, rather than discuss a topic in the abstract. With Shanidar Z and Richard III, a named human at a specific point in time becomes a symbol, a shorthand for a more general social need for authenticity and belonging. We recognize people from the past as 'just like us', and simultaneously recognize ourselves, not just as individuals, but as nations and species; as somehow permanent.

And yet, not all of us find it easy to recognize others. When I peered at the shrunken heads in the Pitt Rivers Museum all those years ago, I was already fascinated by faces. I had been tormented by nightmares as a young child, and in one recurring dream a strange man with a pocket watch had his back to me. When I tapped him on the shoulder – which I was compelled to do in every dream – he would turn around to reveal a face ravaged by the plague.

Unsurprisingly, that stranger's face is memorable to me, even now, whereas others are not. For years I have struggled to know faces, to remember them, to order them in my mind. But I was in my forties before I found out that I have prosopagnosia, or face-blindness, a so-called neurological dysfunction first named (or invented) by the German neurologist Joachim Bodamer in 1947. What difference might prosopagnosia make to the history of the face, and to what the face means in our modern age of facehood? Come with me to my daughter's nursery to find out.

8.
Recognized

It was 5.30 p.m. and I was standing in the corridor of my daughter's nursery. The odour of over-cooked vegetables and over-filled nappies was mixed with those of antibacterial cleanser and perfumed plastic sacks, and I could hear the last sing-song stages of a child's farewell celebration: 'Bye-bye Mabel, Mabel is leaving; Bye-bye Mabel, Mabel is leaving'. As the music tailed off, and over-tired children began to complain, other parents appeared in the corridor, mumbling tired 'Hellos', finishing off calls, rooting through Lost Property for mislaid jumpers, scarves, Lego figures.

All eyes were on the blue metal safety gate that separated the corridor from the nursery proper, where a perky staff member dressed in a yellow tabard appeared. She greeted us all – anonymously, brightly – 'mums and dads' – as a gaggle of children aged three to five appeared, some with snot-green noses, others clinging to sleeves of cardigans and arms of teddies. Somewhere in that sea of unformed, upturned faces was my little girl. But where?

As the safety gate opened and the children surged forward in a throng of giggles, complaints, demands to be fed, wails that they weren't invited to someone's party or had lost their unicorn, a wave of little white girls surged towards me, each body dressed in an identical princess outfit, each face framed with a halo of dark hair. Tiny hands patted at my legs, cooed at my glittery scarf, demanded to know where Millie's baby brother was.

I scanned their faces, trying to remember which princess dress my child had worn that morning, which hair bobbles we had decided on – the purple or the orange? At last, she broke from the crowd and threw her arms around my legs. I put my hand down and cupped her cheek and yes, there she was. Indefinably, absolutely, indivisibly her. I bent down to press my nose against her scalp and to smell that unique scent she had, the one that I could discern from a billion babies the moment she was born. I took her sticky hand and led her out of the nursery with a discreet sigh of relief: I had found her.

There is nothing quite as humbling, as destabilizing, as failing to recognize your own child. Most of the time, when you walk past a colleague or misrecognize someone at a conference, you can say 'oh, I was distracted; I was miles away', and pump their hand enthusiastically, putting it down to absent-mindedness or out-of-context-ness.

But your own child? At nursery? It's not the kind of thing one admits to. I am doing so now, some twenty years later, because I know her face so well, and I have proven my deep, unconditional love, I hope, many times. She is also aware of my affliction; laughs at the fact that it still takes me a few seconds to recognize others; worries that she will inherit it.

Most people are not aware. Like anyone masking, I have learned to 'pass'.

I was five years into my research project on faces before I realized that I had prosopagnosia. I had only a vague understanding of the condition before then, as it isn't well known. The term comes from the classical Greek, *prosop* for 'face'; *agnosia* for 'not knowing'; informally it is called 'face-blindness'.

Think how much we take for granted when it comes to the face – not only about how we judge and assess others, a common theme throughout this book, but also that we will know others by their faces: friends, colleagues, children.

There are levels of prosopagnosia, as we will see, and a few celebrities have recently outed themselves as face-blind – most recently Joanna Lumley and Brad Pitt. In an interview with *GQ* magazine, Pitt recounted how he struggled to remember new people or remember their faces, and feared it made people think he was remote and self-absorbed. When the interviewer tells him that her husband also has prosopagnosia, Pitt was excited. 'Nobody believes me!' he cried. 'I wanna meet another.'

Pitt's fears are natural, and familiar. Because faces are so fundamental to social communication and identity, not recognizing someone can feel like a snub – as perplexing for the person not recognized as for the one who is face-blind. Recognizing people is an expected part of the two-way communication between individuals, groups and institutions. Babies need to recognize caregivers; friends need to recognize allies, and enemies. To some degree this must be part of our human as well as our social evolution, though our early human ancestors would not have needed to remember a fraction of the number of faces we survey today – on this, more later.

The scientific story of prosopagnosia begins, like so many medical developments, with trauma and war. When prosopagnosia was first identified by Joachim Bodamer in 1947, the condition was related to brain damage, that is, *acquired* prosopagnosia. He based his findings on the study of three brain-injured German soldiers, all of whom had problems recognizing faces and even expressions.

If a person has no problems recognizing people before an injury, and then there is a measurable and noticeable decline in face recognition after injury, this indicates a change in brain function. Developmental prosopagnosia, which is not linked to any known cause, is harder to explain, and diagnose.

The term prosopagnosia had made its way into the *Oxford English Dictionary* by 1950, defined as 'agnosia in recognition of physiognomy', but it is still not well understood. Scientific journals continue to debate the causes, and what is specific about recognizing faces as opposed to other categories of objects, like houses or cars.

Most people who study prosopagnosia are psychologists or neuroscientists – a legacy of the mind being reduced to brain (you might remember from earlier chapters that it was once more holistically linked to soul). One of the most prominent of these researchers was the neurologist Oliver Sacks, who himself suffered from face-blindness.

Sacks had a problem remembering places as well as faces. The English neurologist John Hughlings Jackson, best known for his work on epilepsy, described such a case of visual agnosia – for places and faces – in 1872. It's quite common for the two to be associated; for people with face-blindness to also experience place-blindness. Before satnav was common in cars, I used to plaster the dashboard in Post-It notes to navigate from my house in Manchester to Lancaster University, where I worked. I made that journey three times a week, but I could remember nothing about the route; once the Post-It notes fell off, I found myself driving to Liverpool instead.

I can get lost in towns and buildings too; most memorably when I had to attend a full-day's assessment for a job. The test was in Heslington Hall, a large manor house in York owned by the University of York. Ten of us were undertaking a writing test when I left the assessment room to go to the toilet. On my return I couldn't remember the way back to the test. Someone passed me in the corridor and smiled, but I didn't know whether that was one of the candidates or someone being friendly. I finally found the room, but didn't recognize anyone in it. I did recognize the bright-red jacket worn by the assessor, which gave me the confidence to enter.

Place-blindness, like face-blindness, can be both developmental and acquired. Although place-blindness is more common in acquired brain injuries, as developmental experiences they can be seen as a kind of neurological dysfunction. But it is still less embarrassing to be bad at navigating space than it is to forget people entirely. Sacks notes, as Pitt does, that 'my frequent inability to recognise schoolmates would cause bewilderment, and sometimes offense – it did not occur to them (why should it?) that I had a perceptual problem.'

No amount of knowing you have a problem with faces makes it easier to fix – it's not a skill that you can practise, such as riding a bicycle or touch-typing. And so, we move through the world constantly fearing that people's feelings will be hurt, or they'll think we don't value them enough to remember them, or that we are just rude. I moved into a new apartment a year ago, and though I have spoken to the neighbours often and study their faces carefully each time, I cannot lock them into my memory. And so, I look hesitantly at every person I pass on our street who is of a similar age and sex and shape – just in case.

My inability to remember people has not generally been reflected in how I feel about them, but I am more likely to remember the face of an individual who is striking, or familiar, and we will come back to why that might be later.

It is humbling to be 'bad at faces' for all the reasons covered in this book – faces are a sign of identity, of personhood, of emotion and communication; they are special to humans. Our social status, and often our safety, depends on being able to tell one person apart from another. We might identify people through voice and clothes and gait and body language, and even scent. But as we saw in the chapter on photography, being known legally as well as socially by your face has become increasingly significant.

Yet there are many ways we know a person. My fingers can still remember how my little daughter's cheek felt beneath my palm, and I can still bring her childhood scent to mind. Which makes me wonder how far, when unconnected to injury and disease, prosopagnosia might be defined as a social problem rather than a neurological one. In other words, it is only because we are expected to know a face – because our entire society is ordered around facial recognition – that prosopagnosia becomes a problem.

How many people have prosopagnosia? We don't know. Testing isn't widely available and anyway the tests are limited. Brain scans are the most effective way to assess brain activity in relation to facial recognition, and this is done through functional magnetic resonance imaging (fMRI) scans, which we encountered in the previous chapter.

When the neurons of the brain are activated, they need more oxygen from red blood cells, and that movement leads to measurable changes in blood flow. So, fMRI scans light up areas of the brain that are active when we look at faces. The academic study of prosopagnosia uses these images to determine normal standards of facial recognition; it has defined a 'standard' from which some people deviate. At one end of the scale is prosopagnosia and at the other end 'super-recognition' – a term coined at Harvard University as recently as 2009.

The company Super Recognisers International tells us that people with such an ability are 'extraordinary'; that 'the skill cannot be taught – Super Recognisers are born this way'. People with super-recognition can apparently recognize 80 per cent of faces they have seen once before, as compared to 20 per cent in the general population. There are no routine tests for super-recognition or prosopagnosia, but both conditions are supposed to count for 2 per cent of the population – all this really means is that they are the two extremes of the presumed bell curve, with most people landing somewhere in the middle.

The science behind facial recognition reveals something fascinating about how we think the brain works. Since the nineteenth century, and the work of the French physician Paul Broca, who identified a brain area associated with language, scientists have focused on brain regionalization – the idea that different areas of the brain specialize in specific functions. We came across this in the 'Expressed' chapter, and the belief that different emotions originated in specific parts of the brain (e.g. the amygdala used to be known as the 'fear centre').

Now we know that emotions are much more widely distributed across the brain, involving several different networks that work together. But still different parts of the brain are specialized for movement, language, memory, vision, and emotional regulation. In visual processing, for instance, the occipital lobe at the back of the brain plays a role; for more specialized tasks, such as face recognition, the fusiform gyrus in the temporal lobe is important. The whole region is involved in object and face recognition; damage – of the kind identified by Bodamer in the 1940s – results in face-blindness, though cars and colours can still be recognized.

Isn't it odd that a single function can be disrupted while others remain intact? There must be larger networks sustaining everyday cognitive abilities. And the brain does have an extraordinary ability for some parts to 'fill in' for others – there are medical cases of a person surviving, even living well, with just half a brain!

Within the fusiform gyrus sits the fusiform face area (FFA) – identified by the Canadian neuroscientist Justine Sergent in 1992, and named five years later by an American neuroscientist, Nancy Kanswisher. The FFA seems to be particularly important in facial recognition, because it activates when a person looks at a face (the fusiform gyrus more generally is activated when looking at other objects or shapes).

The finding of the FFA backs up the idea that there is something special about faces; that they are so important to humans – through communication and emotional expression, through identity and connection – that they deserve their own brain area. A similar finding was made in the 1960s with other primates – the neuroscientist Charles Gross found that some areas of monkeys' brains responded to the hands of other monkeys, but there was even more activity when they looked at their faces.

Since Gross's work, a great deal of neuroscientific research has been undertaken into the functioning of the brain and the visual cortex. What was once ridiculed – the idea that identifying hands or faces is an activity carried out by key specialist cells – is now widely accepted. So too is the idea that babies have a 'face hunger' from birth, actively seeking faces and face-shaped patterns to stare at – even foetuses might do it, as we found in an earlier chapter.

So, there's no doubt that the brain considers faces important. But here's where things get complicated – the debate has centred in psychology on whether the FFA is *really* unique to faces, or more generally involved in identifying other objects.

And there are more pressing questions. Mike Burton, a Professor of Psychology at the University of York, is frustrated by the debate's narrowness. He is more interested in how we know the faces of others at all – especially faces that are familiar to us.

This is neglected in most prosopagnosia tests, which involve the subject looking at a series of black and white faces presented on a computer screen. One version relies on images of celebrities – Brad Pitt, perhaps, followed by Queen Elizabeth II, Tom Cruise, Elvis Presley, Barack Obama – and tests the viewer on whether they have seen that face before.

This test arguably reveals less about a person's facial processing than their familiarity with Western politics and culture. To some degree, when we see a face, we notice what surrounds it; this is particularly important in iconic and celebrity faces – Elvis's face is harder to recognize without his quiff, Queen Elizabeth's without her crown.

Another limitation of such tests is that we do not usually experience a person's face through a series of static images, but in relation to the other elements that make a person unique: their tone of voice, height, weight, gait, clothes, skin tone and hair. And a face that moves is usually more readable than a face that is still. I have often been bewildered by a new face, only to have that face open its mouth, and invite a flood of recognition.

Many people live with a sense that they are 'good' or 'bad' with faces, without ever being assessed or diagnosed. Which brings us back to Mike Burton's question: what is it about the faces that we know that makes them so familiar?

Instead of testing whether people can recognize well-known figures, Mike and his team study how the brain remembers familiar objects – not just any kitchen, cat, or mother, but rather my kitchen, my cat, or my mother. This highlights a relational aspect of facial recognition that is often left out of any discussion; how we form connections with faces over time, and how we remember familiar faces differently from unfamiliar ones.

Mike's work makes me think about my own experience with prosopagnosia and its connection to familiar faces. I knew my daughter's face by the time she was four, although that face was young and unformed (there's a reason why super-recognizers are better at recognizing adults than children). And I was emotionally connected to my daughter, though I was overwhelmed by the sensory unfamiliarity of the nursery environment. Most of us have had that experience of seeing someone we know in the wrong place, which means we might not recognize them, and it is always harder to notice things when we are stressed and distracted.

These social contexts are more important to the experience of prosopagnosia than focusing on the FFA in isolation. Emotional and sensorial triggers always affect how we see and remember faces. So, while I am sympathetic to calls for prosopagnosia to be regarded as a disability, we need to know more about when and why it happens.

Moreover, people who have sensory overload and other forms of neurological divergence are far more likely to experience prosopagnosia than those who are neurotypical; more than 30 per cent of people with autism also have face-blindness. In fact, nearly 60 per cent of people with a formal diagnosis of prosopagnosia have at least one developmental co-morbidity, such as ADHD or post-traumatic stress disorder (PTSD).

Why hasn't this overlap received more attention? Abilities outside the norm, including prosopagnosia and neurological divergence, tend to be regarded as outliers or disabilities, rather than equally valid but different ways of inhabiting the world. It is simply the case that those on the wrong end of the bell curve don't meet the demands of modern Western society.

Another reason for the lack of join-up is that neuroscientists are rarely experts in neurodivergence. Neuroscience typically focuses on specific brain regions and systems, whereas neurodivergence demands a more holistic and broad-based approach. There is also little funding for the interdisciplinary research that could bridge these gaps.

There is hope; some researchers are beginning to look at how emotional, social and sensory issues contribute to prosopagnosia. This is encouraging because it takes the focus off prosopagnosia as a pathology – and it invites us to see faces and facial recognition as a meaning-making, rather than meaning-reflecting, part of our relationship with others.

To delve further into my own prosopagnosia, Mike Burton introduced me to his colleague Dr David Pitcher, a cognitive neuroscientist working on face perception. David believes we can't study the FFA in isolation; when it comes to perceiving faces, the FFA works with the fusiform body area (FBA) and the extrastriate body area (EBA) to guide our encounters – which suggests we need to update our two-pathway model of visual processing.

The two-pathway model normally used is the ventral, which is responsible for identifying things, and the dorsal, which focuses on spatial awareness – where those things are. Now, David Pitcher and his team have identified a third visual pathway that they believe is unique to human and non-human primates.

This third pathway responds to moving faces as well as bodies, mapping across the whole visual field to help process a range of social cues. It allows us to appreciate the importance of the face for human and to a lesser degree non-human primates; and it offers a holistic perspective on the ways we engage with others. It also allows for faces to be considered alongside other aspects of human interaction – including facial expression, body language, gesture, tone of voice and eye gaze.

This relational, emotional approach to facial recognition helps us to move away from the crude idea – rejected throughout this book – that the face is a thing outside of culture. It might also help explain why we remember some faces more easily than others.

David Pitcher enlists me in a study he is running. He has booked an fMRI machine as part of his investigation into the third pathway – and I am keen to see my brain. I found it nerve-wracking, to sit on an fMRI bed and put in earplugs and put on headphones in the presence of people I hardly knew. Later I say this to David, remarking on how I felt incongruous, dressed like a civilian while others were in white coats. David tells me he doesn't own a white coat, and I realize that my memory must have invented it – a reminder of the power dynamics in situations that involve scientific expertise, equipment and unfamiliar spaces.

As I lie down and look up, a series of images flash on the screen above my head, and I feel suddenly relaxed, far more than I have been in months. I concentrate on the faces of toddlers in red T-shirts clamping plump fingers over giggling mouths and rolling about in nappies, before viewing country roads overhung with dappled leaves, reminding me of growing up in Wales. Then the images are of hands, moving over toy fire engines, pushing cars across carpets, bunching into mouths.

I can hear David through the headphones, but I can't see him or his colleagues. They are sitting behind the glass window which separates his office from the electromagnet that is sending radio waves – some 50,000 times greater than the Earth's magnetic field – through my head. The fMRI is creating slices of my brain as overlaid images that can be viewed and compared to the brains of others – another kind of composite imaging, I think, recalling Francis Galton, whom we met in the chapter on photography.

I wonder what David can see on his screen, and whether the FFA and that third pathway is lighting up as I stare at the children on mine. And I have another unsettling thought – does my brain look normal? It's oddly vulnerable and intimate to have someone look inside your body, seeing what you will never see, and interpreting it in a way that you could not. It reminds me of foetal scanning, which decodes our babies inside our wombs, in ways most of us can never read.

And then, too soon, for apart from these abstract thoughts my brain has been pleasantly quiet, the test ends. 'Was it as bad as you thought?' David asks. I say no, that it was helpful in reducing my brain's usual noise – there was something calming about the rhythmic and insistent hum, the flashing images. I would have stayed longer if I could have. David tells me about another strand of his work, targeting anxiety – but only briefly, as his next study-subject has arrived.

'I will let you know when the results are back,' he says. I expect to wait a couple of weeks; he will need to run the results by medics first, to make sure there's nothing untoward on the scan. It is agreed on the consent forms that if the scan picks up anything pathological – a tumour for example – my doctors and I would be informed. I am appreciative of that. Not all researchers guarantee that they would let you know, and this is a genuine and ongoing ethical challenge for them: do you tell the person being scanned, if the outcome has nothing to do with the test? And what if there is a tumour that cannot be operated on, and the remainder of a person's life will be negatively impacted by knowing that? David reassures me that he has scanned hundreds of people and never found a tumour.

I try to forget about the scan, but I have spent too much time thinking about the brain, and what can go wrong; too many hours reading stories of sudden holes in language that emerge overnight and are revealed to be the products of worms or degeneration. Too much time dwelling on the reasons why a person might cease to recognize faces, and places, from menopausal distraction to dementia and the potential health hazards of aluminium pans.

Then, unexpectedly, when I have almost forgotten about it, David's email appears. And with it, a scanned black and white image. 'Thanks for coming in,' the email says. 'This is a picture of your brain' (fig. 34).

As I stare at the image I feel a variety of sensations. The first is relief. I don't appear to have a tumour; though I don't have the skills or training to read a brain scan and decide that the slightly fuzzy area in the right frontal cortex must be normal.

What are you supposed to feel, I wonder, when confronted by your own interior? I think about those early experiments by the German scientist Wilhelm Conrad Roentgen. In 1895 he discovered how to create images of the body with X-rays that could pass through soft tissues but leave bones and metal visible. One of the earliest images he captured was of his wife Bertha's hand, a wedding ring visible on bony, fleshless fingers. The story goes that on seeing the image, Bertha declared 'I have seen my death', and refused to return to her husband's laboratory.

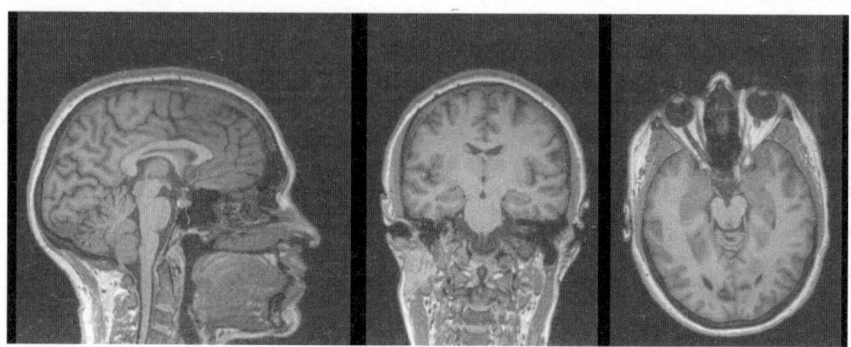

34. 'This is a picture of your brain': an fMRI scan, 2022.

Recognized

My friend Samantha commented on the shape of my brain stem. 'I had no idea it went up so high into the brain,' she said. I hadn't either. Is it supposed to, I wondered, is it always that shape? I discovered, in showing the scan to others, especially those well versed in such images, a self-conscious embarrassment – as if I were handing round holiday snaps that reveal belly rolls and dimply thighs. And yet the same organ I was looking at was somehow responsible for these feelings. I enjoyed imagining my thoughts moving along those material, physical pathways – as if, somehow, that proved I was in charge.

How strange that by mapping something, by seeing it, we can create an illusion of control! Which, after all, is the premise of scientific medicine, and the study of the face.

I showed my brain scan to two more people that week: colleagues at King's College London; an ennobled Professor of Psychiatry and a Professor of English. The psychiatrist has seen many such scans before and jokes that there's something wrong with it. The English professor shares my fascination with the technology that produced it. Another colleague, a neuroscientist, offers to dissect an 'old brain' for me so that I can see the FFA laid bare; he means a brain that has been used for anatomical teaching and has come to the end of its use.

Immediately, I imagine the scent of formaldehyde. It's one thing to see an image of your own brain, alive, but another to see someone else's remains. Or to dig part of it out and see it plop onto the anatomy desk, as David Pitcher recalled seeing during an anatomy lecture. The instructor had wanted to show how quickly life could be snuffed out.

'I sat there,' David said, 'thinking, if that is removed, I would die in three seconds, just like that. Like you're nothing but meat in the end.' I didn't, at the time, notice David's allusion to the Tori Amos song, 'Blood Roses'.

I visit David once more to talk about the scanned images – this time in his office, between visits from his students. David is visibly more relaxed than he had seemed in his lab, without the whirring of machines and the responsibilities attached to the scanning. I sit beside him as he pulls up on his desktop computer several images of my brain. Together we move through its slices, from the top, the back, the side.

With a forefinger, David outlines the hippocampus, the amygdala, the areas we associate with emotion, the clearly delineated frontal cortex for decision-making. I say something about the amygdala hijacking the frontal cortex when we are anxious, and David winces. 'It's not always clear where the impetus originates,' he says, 'or what is hijacking what.'

Then he pulls up brightly coloured images of my brain, with sections lit up to reflect the firing of my neurons. 'That's when you were looking at the hands and faces of children,' he says, pointing out the FFA, lit up now in red. And there is the third pathway, an area of activity extending beyond the FFA, which David and his team relate to sociability. It too is lit up, as is the front of my brain – the prefrontal cortex, active in tasks involving complex processing. When you're seeing faces, and hands, and places, the prefrontal cortex helps put it all in context.

I had half-wondered if, because of my prosopagnosia, the FFA wouldn't fire up when I looked at faces, but apparently it does; the FFA is often active, too, in people who are blind. Some fMRI scans of people with autism do show less activation in the FFA than in neurotypical people. But the strongest response to faces in people with autism is activated in regions typically reserved for objects.

Does that mean people with autism do not feel so strongly about faces? Or does it mean that they feel more strongly about objects? Maybe it just means that neurodivergent people can have different priorities in communication.

We are back to the limited research on connections between faces and neurodivergence. We tend to speak about people with autism having 'difficulties' in reading the emotions of others, but this is an oversimplification: there are different manifestations of autism.

One common, but not universal, phenomenon found in fMRI scans is that people with autism have less activation in the FFA when looking at human faces than when looking at animal faces. Which is interesting, because some people with autism prefer relationships with non-verbal animals such as dogs. Perhaps this is because dogs are more straightforward about how they communicate than humans.

In neurotypical people, face-specific regions of the brain are also proportionally larger in adults than they are in children, which suggests that the change is caused by social experience and habituation – that we learn to hone our facial recognition as we age.

That doesn't seem to happen in people with autism, and autistic people are less likely to see faces in material objects, such as plugs or street signs, a phenomenon called pareidolia. This term, like prosopagnosia, comes from classical Greek (*para*, meaning 'alongside' or 'instead of', and *eidolon*, 'shape' or 'image'). Some studies have suggested that pregnant women are more likely than others to see faces in things, as though their brains are readying for new neural connections with their babies. And babies, as we saw earlier, are always searching for face patterns.

Of course, perceiving faces isn't the same as *knowing* faces – though both seem entangled with our broader, and ongoing, neuro-social development. Some of us will never be good with faces, but we are proficient at different ways of knowing the people who matter to us.

Even the best brain scans tell us nothing about what it's like to live with face-blindness. They can't tell the degree to which I have prosopagnosia or describe the emotional or social impact of not remembering faces. At best, they can measure if there is activity in my brain. It's not their job to judge the impact of my failure to recognize a person at a social or an emotional level. Which remains awkward.

David laughs and tells me I don't seem awkward. And anyway, how often is it a problem?

'Let's imagine,' he says, 'that you're one degree of standard deviation away from the mean.' David is referring to the bell curve of facial recognition – which is a common way to plot any trait or ability. At the centre, or the top of the bell, we have the average or mean that most people are clustered around. A small standard deviation, such as one degree, is average. At two or more standard deviations we find prosopagnosiacs and super-recognizers.

'Does it matter if you are one standard deviation away from the mean?' David asks. 'After all, how many people do we really need to recognize in our lifetimes?'

Far more than we used to, is the answer to that. Our earliest ancestors would have needed to know who was in their group and who was outside it. For centuries, our communities might have included fewer than 100 people with faces to remember. In the 1420s most people would have known the faces of family, neighbours and other villagers, and might have seen images of their ruler, their gods, perhaps some saints. By the 1920s, photography, advertising, cinemas and television flooded the world with faces.

Today we 'know' hundreds of people we might never meet in person. We encounter online, and in images, thousands more people than our ancestors would have done. Some 56 per cent of the world's population – 4.4 billion people – live in cities. Human populations have expanded exponentially, from perhaps one billion people in 1800 to an anticipated 10 billion by 2100. Millions of faces are beamed in our direction over our lifetimes – many more, surely, than the average brain could ever remember.

Mike Burton and his colleague Rob Jenkins ran an experiment with twenty-five students that suggested that a brain might know 5,000 faces. To qualify as 'knowing' a face, participants had to recognize it in two different photographs, from a gallery of images that included Barack Obama and Tom Cruise. Famous people in Western culture in other words, the knowledge of which is generational as well as geographical.

The actual range of facial recognition was between 1,000 to 10,000 faces. Where do you fit on that scale? These individual variations are important – some people are naturally better at faces, just as they are better at gymnastics or mathematics; there is a bell curve for everything. But the ways we experience prosopagnosia might vary.

If it's tiresome not to know the faces of people you ought to know, what about thinking you know the faces of people when you don't? Many of us have seen a famous person on the street and thought we knew them – we have seen their faces so often that they feel familiar. It's common, too, for us to think someone reminds us of someone else – a dead ringer or a doppelgänger.

To wit, I have carried on whole conversations with people who turned out to be someone else. There was the time I joined a woman for breakfast in a hotel, thinking she was my companion from the previous day's conference. We talked for a while before it emerged that she was someone else entirely. In my defence, she looked similar to the woman at the conference: white, middle-aged, blonde hair, with average features. If people's faces are distinctive, if there is something extraordinary about them, I do remember them. But that distinctive thing is as likely to be their hair, the way they laugh or walk, as it is their face.

Even distinctive people can be forgettable, when they are in the wrong place. When I had to rehome a kitten, a colleague sent her friend Lizzy round to see the cat. I asked Lizzy how she knew my colleague, only to be met by a look of confusion. Lizzy was also my colleague, and her office was opposite mine; we had spoken in the corridor several times. That experience was harder to explain, for Lizzy is unusually beautiful. Perhaps, following Mike Burton's theory, this was simply a lack of familiarity. I had only just joined the department and hadn't seen Lizzy's face often enough for it to be familiar. Fortunately, Lizzy had heard of prosopagnosia, so I was able to explain the problem, though the excuse sounded hollow.

Distinctiveness and familiarity intersect in interesting ways. I tell David Pitcher about the time I was expecting a visit from a man I was dating. When his car pulled up, I waved and called 'Hello'. Then he got out of the car and went to the boot. As I watched him move, I had the distinct impression something wasn't right. I stared at the man: *was* that my boyfriend?

I had no idea; it was like staring at a maths puzzle and waiting for the numbers to slot into place, only they didn't. I looked at the car and realized that it wasn't a grey BMW, and the registration plate was wrong. Its driver was still looking at me in confusion when the man I *was* dating pulled up in his car. Pretending nothing was wrong, I waved again and said 'Hello'.

'Maybe the man lied in his dating profile,' David mused. 'Was it a new relationship?' When I said no, I had been dating him for two years, David leant back in his chair. 'OK, I revise my initial statement,' he said. 'That's the kind of story I hear from people who are two or three degrees away from the mean.'

I puzzled over this for a while. The boyfriend was familiar to me, but he wasn't distinctive – he resembled many middle-aged men who lived in the same part of England that their ancestors had for generations. He had mannerisms that were particular to him, such as the way he turned out his feet when he walked, and how he patted down the hair that stuck up at his forehead, but his face never seemed to stick.

Familiar faces do not normally have to be distinctive to be remembered; they are familiar because we see them from many different angles in a wide range of contexts. They are also usually invested with emotional meanings – mothers stare at their newborns in wonder and love as they memorize the lines of their face; lovers stare into one another's eyes intoxicated by oxytocin. Some faces are both familiar and distinctive: Brad Pitt is commonly used in prosopagnosia tests for this reason. Familiarity for most people comes from the number of movies Pitt has been in – but what makes his face distinctive?

That's a difficult question for the prosopagnosiac, because it involves describing a person's face. The best I can do is to say Brad Pitt has a slightly snubbed nose and crinkly eyes; if I picture him in my mind, I see his face in motion – specifically doffing his cowboy hat in *Thelma & Louise* (like David's white coat, I might have made this up).

So, I asked AI to describe what is distinctive about the actor's face. With the enthusiasm of a teenager describing their first crush, it gushed that Pitt had a chiselled jawbone, high cheekbones, piercing eyes, facial symmetry, a 'youthful yet rugged look', versatile facial expressions and golden hair. A remarkably generic and similar description is given of George Clooney, which is unsurprising since both actors fall into a classically Hollywood version of male attractiveness.

Staying with male actors for consistency, I asked AI to tell me what is distinctive about Adrien Brody's face. Its reply was that Brody has a long angular face, a prominent nose, deep-set eyes, full lips, high cheekbones and a slim build. Brody's attractiveness, and his distinctiveness, comes from that unusual combination of features, which also makes him familiar – I would have much less difficulty describing his face to someone than Pitt's face, or Clooney's. But again, I picture his face in motion – and emotion – a face in feeling, rather than static; and as a similarly prosopagnosiac friend pointed out, he has the most expressive eyebrows!

In art and entertainment, the combined qualities of distinctiveness and familiarity can be as important to casting as they are to caricature. In action movies, directors and producers want faces that are easily recognizable as tropes as much as individual actors. This happens across a range of art forms, and it is why villains – such as Richard III, whom we met in the previous chapter – are often given sharp features, scars or thin lips as a shorthand for cruelty.

Distinctiveness is not always the same thing as attractiveness, but it marks a person out as memorable; this is one reason why I find the homogenization of beauty on Instagram so unnerving. But perhaps we need to think more about distinctiveness and familiarity, together with place, emotions and memory, when we research the causes and effects of developmental prosopagnosia – at least if we want to understand why people might recognize faces differently.

And I say *differently*, because face-blindness is not necessarily a defect. We might prioritize vision as the most important sense and faces as the essence of individualism, but there are other ways of knowing a person.

Those with developmental prosopagnosia do not tend to have difficulties reading emotions; I'm highly attuned to changes in a person's expression and demeanour. Nine times out of ten I can read a misalignment between what a person is saying and what they are feeling, and my intuitive sense of a person is far more important to me than what their face looks like.

Of course, intuition has no scientific basis (yet); neuroscientist friends tell me that my intuition can be reduced to the microexpressions I am unconsciously reading on the faces of others, but I am not convinced.

Knowledge about a person comes from our body, as well as our brain – we might explain it in terms of pattern recognition or subconscious processing, but it seems to be a social sense as much as a psychological one.

Faces are part, but not the totality, of what makes us recognizable to others. In research terms we are only scratching the surface of what prosopagnosia means as a cultural and social phenomenon, let alone a neurological or psychological one. It is too easy for ways of being and knowing to be locked into systems and parts of the body as dysfunctions, rather than honoured as individual and evolving ways of experiencing the world.

Because of our focus on the brain and on neuroscience, the idea that there is only one way to look at and process faces, and that everything else is on a spectrum of abnormality, is spoken about as truth. But it is a product of history.

I am making this claim about developmental rather than acquired prosopagnosia for one simple reason – in acquired prosopagnosia, as with Joachim Bodamer's injured soldiers, damage to the brain usually disrupts an already learned way of processing faces. That learning develops as our brains evolve in relation to the world around us, and alongside other sensory ways of perceiving. If we are neurologically divergent, or we have childhood trauma (the two often being related), or if we are visually impaired, we might develop other perceptive skills, ones not so reliant on faces. And if we want to hold on to the primary importance of the brain, we can see those perceptive skills as a neuroplastic adaptation.

Faces are especially important to humans, but some animals

recognize themselves, as we saw in Darwin's experiments with his infant son Doddy and the orangutan. Many animals also show same-species recognition – that is, they seem to know one another; sheep do, and pigs, monkeys and apes, cattle, dogs, pigeons and even, delightfully, honeybees and ants.

Their recognition isn't always visual. It can be based on smell, sound and behaviour, and generally a combination of them. Ants, for instance, use their antennae to smell, touch and communicate; each ant releases a compound that is detected, and recognized, based on odour. We might say that ants have scenthood, rather than facehood.

Humans might not have antennae, or such a precise sense of smell, but people with face-blindness are more likely to pay attention to factors beyond facial appearance – scent, movement, gait, clothes, hairstyle, tone and timbre of voice, as well as that innate energetic quality that is impossible to put into words, but which can make ugly people beautiful, and vice versa.

What about people with visual impairments? I asked my friend and project collaborator Annalyn Bell Wiens, who has been blind since she was two years old. She tells me she can assess a person's weight, mass, height, mood, intentions and identity, if they are in the same room. 'It's voices,' she says. 'The kind of extra weight on the voice, the sound and pitch and everything. To me, that's no different to just looking at someone's face.'

Annalyn dreams about people, but their bodies are vague, and their faces have no centre, 'it's just a circle, with a void inside'. And this is fine, she says, because in many ways, 'the whole body is a face'.

What would happen to our understanding of faces, and prosopagnosia, if we thought about facial recognition in a more sensorial and emotional way – and considered how we recognize others over a person's lifespan? We know that adults are better at knowing faces than children, and we presume that this is because our skills improve as we grow.

Many of us, in later life, unlearn that skill; it is no coincidence that knowing faces is one of the earliest things an infant can do, and that unlearning faces is linked to ageing and a loss of connection. Alzheimer's and dementia mean that our ties of social connection start to unravel along with our ability to remember or decode faces and bodies at all.

I think about the fear and confusion of my Grandma Rose when I visited her nursing home with my son; after a long journey he had fallen asleep in his pushchair, his head tilting forward in such a way that a curly mop of blond hair obscured his face. 'What is it?' Grandma Rose asked in confusion as she pointed at him. 'What *is* it?'

Maybe we should think about prosopagnosia less in relation to super-recognition, and more alongside other ways of knowing the face – such as pareidolia. Seeing faces in things could serve an evolutionary purpose in making us more attuned to potential threats; it is also a kind of pattern recognition linked to creativity and innovation. You may remember that it is also common in new mothers, who are particularly sensitive to the faces of their babies. There are both collective and individual imaginings of pareidolia, too – think of the 'man in the moon', the face of Jesus, which has appeared in trees, cloud formations and even on toast – or old Polonius persuaded by Hamlet into imagining a camel, then a weasel, then a whale, in the shape of a cloud.

Some associations of pareidolia are negative; it has been described in episodes of schizophrenia and psychosis, as well as anxiety and paranoia. People who have experienced trauma might project difficult memories and emotions onto things in ways that make them feel ever more disconnected from other people.

These complex entanglements between the brain and the body, the face and the world, are important reminders that we are biologically as well as culturally wired to find ourselves in others, and that faces are social as much as individual organs. Our recognition of faces – like the face itself – changes throughout our lives; it is acquired and lost, inherited, learned, developed and modified. It can never be reduced just to the brain, since it is part and parcel of our framework of social and sensory relationships.

The identification of prosopagnosia as a neurological problem tells us more about the progress of scientific medicine – for good and ill – than anything else. Since the 1800s, the body has been taken apart for examination and classified under ever-smaller, more clearly defined systems and specialities – mind and body, circulatory and respiratory, psychiatry, cardiology, dermatology, neurology. We have made significant advances in how we understand illness and disease, but we are also experiencing higher levels of mental illness, anxiety and depression than ever. Lacking comfort, we are a dis-eased society.

Along with medical advances comes risk – and paradoxes. As we saw in an earlier chapter, the face is now viewed, in medicine and surgery, in beauty and the cosmetics industry, as a part of the body to be improved and enhanced in pursuit of happiness or a better life.

In the early twenty-first century, this line of thought arrived at a logical conclusion: faces could even be transplanted. We could take one face, damaged beyond repair, and replace it with another from a dead body; from someone who had agreed to donate other, more conventionally transplanted organs, such as the heart, the liver, the lungs.

The first face transplant in the world took place in France in 2005, which effectively redefined the human face: it was no longer a collection of different structures, including skin, muscles, bones and sensory tissues, but a single organ, which could be passed from one person to another.

Think about what this means. Given the face's cultural significance as the unique identifier of a person, as we have seen repeatedly in this book, what might face transplants have done to our idea of facehood? And who is being recognized when we look at a transplanted face? Let's find out in the following chapter.

9.

Transplanted

In August 2013, Robert Chelsea was driving on the freeway in Los Angeles when his car started to overheat. Smoke billowed from the bonnet, and he pulled over onto the hard shoulder. Moments later, his car was rammed by a drunk driver with such force that it burst into flames. Robert suffered horrific injuries in that crash. His face and body were badly burned, and he lost part of his face and tongue. He spent the next six months in a coma, and the following eighteen months in hospital, where he underwent more than thirty surgeries. Six years later, at the age of sixty-eight, Robert became the first African American, and the oldest person to date, to receive a face transplant (fig. 35).

I first met Robert in April 2022, after speaking to him several times on Zoom. We had been in touch since 2019, when I started working on my project Interface (then called AboutFace), a UKRI-funded study of the history and ethics of face transplants. My research question at that time had been straightforward: Why aren't face transplants available in the United Kingdom?

The U.K. had pioneered facial-reconstruction work during the twentieth century and looked likely to undertake the first face transplant in 2004. So, it was puzzling that face transplants had been done in other countries – France, the U.S., Spain, China – but not the U.K. Was it, as some surgeons claimed, because of red tape, narrow-mindedness and a decline in the innovative drive that used to characterize British science? Or was it due to something else?

Over the next five years, I interviewed most of the people involved in the history of face transplants in the U.K. and internationally. I met several patients who had received face transplants, and their

Transplanted

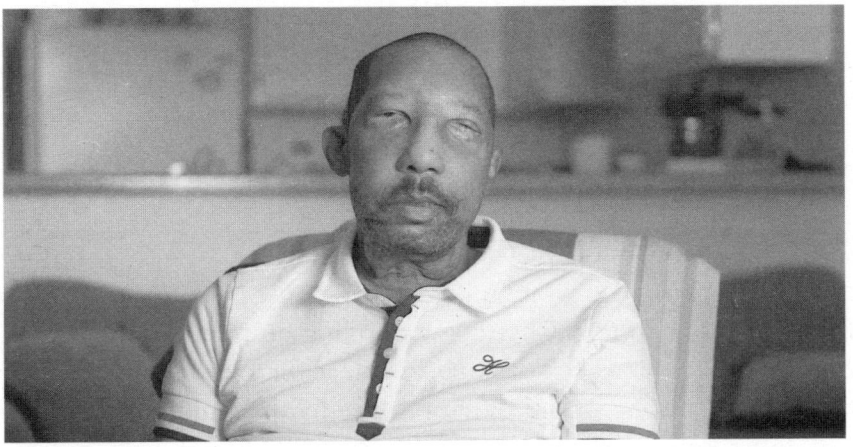

35. Lol Crawley, Robert Chelsea with his transplanted face, 2022.

caregivers. I began to worry for the well-being and future of face-transplant recipients like Robert, who were financially unsupported in countries such as the U.S. that have a commercial healthcare system.

I worried, too, that mistakes from the past were being repeated – that innovation could slide into exploitation, and ethical lines could get blurred. I discovered that treating the face as an 'organ', removing it from its emotional, psychological, social and cultural meanings, came at a considerable cost.

Throughout this book we have seen how important the face has become for individual and social identity, as well as the notion of personhood. We've seen how portrait painting made faces into markers of individualism, how photography made portraying faces democratic, but also vulnerable to surveillance. We've discussed how cosmetic surgery promised to perfect faces as part of the consumer project, and recognition technology track them. And we have observed how technologies of the face are repeatedly shaped and influenced by outdated ideas about race, gender and deviance. Now, with face transplants, we're witnessing the ultimate commodification of the face – literally turning it into something that can be removed, transported and installed on someone else.

How successful is medicine at separating the face from its emotional moorings? And what is the cost? These questions were in my mind as I sat across from Robert in the small, neat living room of his apartment in Pasadena, California, preparing to interview him for my documentary about face transplants. My brother, the cinematographer Lol Crawley, had agreed to help – he lived nearby. So, he borrowed equipment from Paramount Studios and turned up with three trusted crew members, setting me on a journey that has been simultaneously the most rewarding and challenging of my academic career.

Robert is used to being filmed. He's had considerable media attention since his transplant, most of which has focused – as face-transplant reporting generally does – on the miraculous nature of the procedure. We are, as a society, remarkably keen to learn about medical breakthroughs and brilliant surgeons, no matter that medicine has had its share of failures: infected blood, toxic cough syrup, unnecessary breast operations, botched heart surgery, stolen organs, murderous GPs, syphilis injections. We must believe in medical breakthroughs and brilliant surgeons. Otherwise, how would we willingly lie anaesthetized while someone wields a knife over our bodies?

But this faith in face transplants as a medical miracle sits oddly alongside our growing anxiety about faces and identity. We are a culture obsessed with facial recognition, worried about deepfakes, concerned about authenticity in an age of filters and digital manipulation. Yet once the first face transplant took place, we worried less about the identity politics, and – as often happens in the history of medicine – many of the ethics fell by the wayside.

I'm not an anti-vaxxer or a Big Pharma conspiracy theorist, and this isn't a tirade against Western medicine. I see myself as a critical friend, asking questions about systems of care rather than pointing the finger at individual practitioners. And I don't believe that emotion can be left out of medicine – even if it were governed by robot surgeons – technological innovations are filled with bias in training, data and design, as we have seen repeatedly throughout this book.

There's an inevitable imbalance of power between a patient needing help and the doctor giving it, especially when variables such as ethnicity, gender and age come into play. And that is before we critique what 'need' means, as we did in our chapter on perfecting the face.

Surgeons have emotions too – and most of them care about their patients. Most well-known surgeons advance in U.S.-style healthcare systems because they have a will to succeed, to innovate, to prove themselves. Medical breakthroughs happen because of the emotional ideal of progress. It's also the case, unfortunately, that some treatments turn out to be a bad idea: cocaine, fentanyl, vaginal meshes, lobotomies, thalidomide. It's a balancing act.

Some parts of the body carry more emotional meaning than others – hearts, hands and faces. We can't usually see hearts, which have their own intensely rich cultural and emotional history. For centuries they've been linked to the soul, to identity. But we can feel and hear them. Donor relatives have wanted to put their ears to recipients' chests, to hear the heartbeat of their lost person, or to lay their hands on it to feel the heart beating beneath their palm. Transplanted hearts can and do provoke strong emotional responses.

But hands and faces we can see. In transplantation, that visibility raises the stakes, and the emotional meanings. And nothing is more visible, more looked at, more unavoidable, than the face.

Which brings us back to the special status of the face in human history. Remember how portrait painters learned to capture not just likeness but character? How photographers discovered that faces could tell stories about entire societies? How cosmetic surgeons promised to unlock happiness through facial perfection? Each of these developments contributed to what I've been calling 'facehood' as a characteristic of modern society – the idea that a single face is linked to a named and identifiable person.

Face transplants represent the logical endpoint of this process. If faces are truly central to identity, then surely changing your face changes who you are? But if faces are just functional tools for eating, drinking and speaking, then why not replace them like any other body part?

Some face transplants aim to rectify symptoms of disease, conditions such as neurofibromatosis, in which non-cancerous tumours grow in the nerves. More often face transplants are offered after violent attacks, work accidents, self-inflicted gunshot wounds, car crashes – to people who have already experienced considerable trauma.

It's also common for face-transplant recipients to have lived with their injured face for several years before receiving the face of another person. You will have at least three faces during your lifetime as a face-transplant recipient: the face you were born with, your damaged face and the face of a stranger.

Robert told me about the day in August 2013 when his car burst into flames. He holds no ill-will against the driver, even though he already had three DUI convictions and has never contacted Robert to apologize. An extremely religious man, Robert sees everything that was set in motion on that day, from the accident to his rehabilitation and transplant, as a gift from God. He's especially grateful to his rescuer, a passer-by who pulled over, dragged him from the flames and thereby saved his life.

'He grabbed my arm,' Robert said, gesturing at his forearms with a hand that has lost several fingers to amputation, 'but the skin on my arm was melting.'

During Robert's eighteen-month recovery in hospital, staff kept mirrors away from him, as is common with facial injuries. But one day he was wheeled in a chair past a stainless-steel cabinet, and he caught sight of his reflection. He asked the nurse to wheel him back. 'I looked like a Halloween mask,' he said.

Robert's lips and the skin around his mouth had been burned away, leaving his teeth bared and exposed. He couldn't eat easily, or drink without a straw. He couldn't talk clearly or be understood. He couldn't kiss his daughter's cheek, which is what he missed most of all.

This is where the promise of face transplantation becomes most seductive. It offers to give back to the face its social meanings and uses. It also means you're more likely to be able to walk down the street without abuse; some people can be unkind to those who look different, who are 'disfigured'.

The traditional treatment for facial damage and burns is surgical reconstruction, using skin grafts from the patient's own body – taken from a person's thigh or back. This is relatively risk-free treatment. Skin responds quickly to anything foreign – think about how quickly our skin heals after a small cut or bee sting. But if we have other people's skin and tissue rather than our own, as happens in face transplants, then high doses of immunosuppressant drugs are needed to prevent rejection. And those drugs also reduce the patient's normal immune response to other risks, from colds and flu to cancers.

Balanced against the risks of immunosuppressants are the limited aesthetic results of surgical reconstruction. Skin grafts can give faces a patchwork appearance, and the skin feels tight. Burn victims need regular adjustment surgeries, and skin from a thigh is just not the same as skin from lips or eyelids.

Robert's reconstructed face was often stared at by strangers. He was called a freak, a man without a face. But when he was mocked in the street, he made the effort to speak, with his compromised voice, to bullies, and to educate them about the effects of burns. He refused to hide away. He hadn't planned on having any more surgery. He just wanted to get on with his life.

Until he got a call from a man he had never met: Bohdan Pomahac. Bohdan is a leading plastics surgeon with an extraordinary background. Born in Czechoslovakia (now the Czech Republic) in 1971, he emigrated to the U.S. in 1996; there he was so committed to becoming a leading plastic surgeon that he offered to work at Brigham and Women's Hospital in Boston without pay. His interviewer was sufficiently impressed that he offered Bohdan a job, at which Bohdan excelled – and went on to lead the maxillofacial unit.

To date, Bohdan has carried out ten face transplants, including one retransplant when the face failed. The only other surgeon to have done a retransplant is the French surgeon Laurent Lantieri. Today, Bohdan leads the Face Transplant Program at Yale University.

He recently won a multimillion-dollar grant from the Department of Defense to continue his work in face transplants, and to standardize the field of VCA – which stands for vascularized composite allografts, and refers to a specific kind of transplant, involving skin, tissue and bone from a donor. There are several kinds of VCA – hands, penises, wombs, abdominal walls – some of which, like faces, are visible and emotional.

Specialists like Bohdan are the figureheads for this surgery, but they don't work alone – they need multidisciplinary teams of fellow surgeons, anaesthetists, prosthetists, psychologists, immunologists, nurses and physiotherapists. Of the many face-transplant surgeons I've interviewed, Bohdan is among the most thoughtful and pragmatic, driven by the desire to improve life for his patients but limited by the privatized healthcare system in the U.S.

Not all surgeons are ethically minded, especially in countries where competition for funding means that innovative surgery goes hand in hand with personal gain. Leading doctors are referred to, in the media, in books and in conference programmes, as 'rock stars' or 'rock docs'. Sometimes, if you pay more for conference tickets, you can eat breakfast in the same room as them.

This celebrity culture around surgeons echoes something we've seen throughout our exploration of faces: the way in which individual faces become brands, symbols, commodities. Think about how portrait painters competed to capture the faces of the powerful, or how photographers turned faces into icons of beauty or suffering. Now surgeons compete to be associated with the most dramatic facial transformations.

Bohdan had heard about Robert from a fellow surgeon who attended such a conference. With Robert's permission, his details were shared, and so Bohdan gave him a call. He proposed that Robert undergo a face transplant – that he receive a face from a dead donor so he could have lips again, so he could eat and drink properly, protect his mouth from flies, restore basic anonymity when he walked down the street.

Notice what Bohdan offered: not beauty, not perfection, but

invisibility. This is the first thing that people with facial injuries talk to me about when they discuss wanting a face transplant. They don't want to improve on nature or look more attractive. They want to look acceptable, normal enough simply to be invisible – which says a lot about how life is for people with facial difference.

This removal of social stigma has been one of the main reasons face transplants are offered to patients. Surgeons refer to face transplants as 'life-enhancing' rather than life-saving. The two main differences between face transplants and solid-organ transplants (hearts, lungs, livers) are that faces are visible, and you probably won't die without a new face.

Because they are experimental surgeries – only fifty have been carried out globally to date, and long-term data is still being gathered; they are not funded by insurance companies in the US, but rather supported as experimental treatments, primarily by the Department of Defense, which aims to assess whether they are a viable treatment for wounded veterans.

As we saw in an earlier chapter, war tends to produce changes in medicine – either because there are more damaged bodies in need of surgery, which rushes through novel treatments (often, with a higher tolerance for risk), or because it encourages surgeons to experiment.

The medical aspects of face transplantation are complex but straightforward. First, a dead donor of the same sex and reasonably similar age must be found with a matching blood type and compatible tissue antigens. To ensure a good result, the anatomy and size of the donor face should be as similar as possible to the recipient's underlying structure. The colour of the face isn't medically but is socially important, though an ethnic match usually produces better tissue compatability.

Once the donor face has been secured and their family agrees to donate it (which is by no means assured, because faces are so emotional), it must be removed from its original body. In some countries, the fact that the surgery is life-enhancing rather than life-saving means that surgeons must wait until almost every other organ being donated is removed. Then they can get to work detaching the face while another team prepares the recipient to receive it, stripping off the skin, tissue and muscles that are to be replaced.

The window between detaching the face from the donor and re-establishing it on a new body is four hours. Skin, muscles and other tissues are extremely sensitive to oxygen deprivation. Given how rare donor faces are, the stakes are high – within that timeframe the face must be packaged, transported (perhaps by aeroplane), brought into the operating room and attached to the recipient. Can you imagine how tense that situation must be?

During the time that the donor face was being harvested, another surgical team will have been rushing too – stripping the recipient's own face to prepare their body for the transplant. Sometimes bones and even jaws containing teeth need to be connected, using plates and screws, and surgeons use microscopes to connect the arteries, nerves and veins. Once blood flows through the transplanted face, any remaining muscles and nerves are connected, and the skin and soft tissues sewn together.

The patient will have been put on immunosuppressants before the surgery, and, after the transplant, immunologists work with that patient to tailor the medication regimen. They monitor for rejection, tweaking the medications as necessary to support recovery. Nursing staff look after the patient, usually mediating between the surgeons, the family and the individual. Physiotherapists help a patient learn how to use a new mouth and tongue, new cheeks and eyelids. Depending on the extent of the graft, the patient relearns blinking, smiling, eating, drinking, talking, chewing, cleaning their teeth – things most of us take for granted.

Face transplants are risky, rare and experimental. Most people I speak to think they're still science fiction – they might remember the Hollywood movie *Face/Off* (1997), part of the rich history of transplant horrors that betray popular fears of transplants, from Mary Shelley's novel *Frankenstein* (1818) to the movie *The Hands of Orlac* (1924).

Robert had never heard of face transplants when he got that call from Bohdan. His first instinct was to refuse. He'd been through enough surgical treatments, pain and uncertainty to last anyone a lifetime. Robert has an exceptionally strong support network – his daughter Ebony, his godson Ricky, his pastor, the church where he's an elder – and he talked it over with them. Would the risk be worth it? He had limited functionality of his face, to be sure, but otherwise, apart from lingering damage caused by the accident, he was well.

Was it worth running the risks of surgery (rejection, infection, death), as well as those of the medications – especially since a transplanted face is estimated to last just ten years? This figure is speculative – it comes from the world of solid-organ transplants, and we don't honestly know. Kidneys are supposed to last ten-plus years, but the longest reported has been fifty-two. For hearts the average is 12.5 years, and the record is almost forty. Others fail immediately after being implanted.

There isn't yet enough evidence to know the true longevity of transplanted faces, and not all deaths of face-transplant recipients are reported as such. This reflects the lack of information known early on about solid-organ transplants – it takes time for a speciality to become standardized. So, in the meantime, face-transplant recipients are told ten years.

What will those ten years be like? A recipient will have multiple acute rejection episodes during their life; most of these can be managed by amending the dosage of the medication, by flushing out the system with high levels of prednisone – but not always. And there are financial and medical costs for taking all those medications.

When Bohdan called again, he and Robert kept talking. Robert's daughter Ebony wasn't keen. She couldn't understand why he would take any chances – hadn't he been through enough? Hadn't he tempted fate already? Why would he want to endure so much more pain and risk – was it for vanity?

It was Ebony's mother, Robert's ex-wife, who got her on board. She told Ebony about the flies that entered Robert's mouth when he walked down the road. 'This is about health,' she told Ebony, when it was clear that Robert wanted to proceed. But is it?

This remains the big ethical question in the field. How can we take healthy patients and subject them to such risks when the benefits aren't clear? Patients are often asked to fill in standard questionnaires, but these are designed by clinicians to measure function, not feeling. Without involving patients in their design, the deeper emotional meanings of living with a face transplant are easily lost.

In 2022 I held a Policy Lab with several face-transplant surgeons at King's College London, to talk about the questions that were being asked. They agreed that standards of care weren't consistent enough, that the patient's needs weren't being centred, that we didn't really know, yet, how to evaluate face transplants. Articles were published, collaborations secured, more funding won by the surgeons to create better outcomes. Time will tell if it's a success; the will is there, but healthcare systems around the world are so separate, and surgeries are so governed by a clinic's own ethical, legal and financial demands, that change is slow.

How do we decide whether face transplants are successful? Well, we need to talk to patients and their families, to find out whether the results are what they expected; we need to learn whether individuals who took the traditional reconstructive route had better or worse outcomes, we need to keep talking to patients – not just immediately after the surgery, but throughout the remainder of their lives.

Surgeons might ask, 'Can you drink with a straw?' Psychologists, 'Are you satisfied with your appearance?' But hospitals could also ask patients what questions matter most to them—how they make sense of their new face, and what it means to look in the mirror now. Caregivers might be asked, 'How do you feel about your father's or daughter's transplant?' The donor family, too, what it means to see a familiar face on someone new. The recipient won't look exactly like the donor, but other connections live on.

These questions aren't ordinarily asked by surgical teams. In surgery, the transplant is a physical fix that offers a dramatic before-and-after. We've seen throughout this book how powerful and enduring such transformation stories are – from the marketing of cosmetic surgery to historical reconstructions that promise to show us what people 'really looked like'.

Moreover, surgeons don't consider such questions their responsibility; after all, it's not part of their training and there are interdisciplinary teams whose job it is to consider patients' mental health. But here's the thing: psychology teams in the same hospital work within its own hierarchies and ambitions. When a procedure boosts the hospital's reputation or funding, it's hard to stay fully critical. There's quiet pressure not to ask awkward questions – the same pressures that can make it difficult for any medical team to publish negative outcomes. Careers, reputations and funding are all intertwined. Patients don't usually want to criticize or complain either; they worry about being seen as ungrateful, a 'bad patient'.

In 2008, Maria Siemionow, one of the very few female surgeons in the field of facial transplantation, made the case to the *Annals of Plastic Surgery* that the face should be redefined as an organ. If they did not stretch the boundaries of the definition specifically to include faces, faces would have to be bundled in somehow with those other organs that surgeons already had permission to transplant – defined as just 'skin' perhaps? But wouldn't it be more 'degrading' if faces were simply called 'skin'?

The U.S. finally expanded its definition of human organs to include all forms of VCA (Vascularized Composite Allografts), and the face became defined as an organ in 2014. This shift in nomenclature made it ethically easier to detach a face from a donor body; it also attempted to detach the physicality of the face from its uniqueness. It's a perfect example of how language shapes reality. By calling faces 'organs', medicine made them seem more like livers or kidneys – useful but replaceable parts rather than fundamental aspects of human identity.

Is it practical, or achievable, or desirable, to think of the face as an organ? What happens then to its symbolic and emotional status?

These questions take us back to my original research question: Why has no face transplant been undertaken in the United Kingdom to date? As matters currently stand, I don't believe a face transplant will ever be undertaken in the U.K. – not simply because there's a lack of sufficiently wounded patients (we don't have the gun culture and the ballistic injuries that the U.S. has), but because the results have been of variable quality, and there's a high mortality rate.

These are different reasons to those that drove the Royal College of Surgeons to reject face transplants in 2004. At that time, face transplants lay in the future, and it seemed that Peter Butler from London's Royal Free Hospital might undertake the world's first. Butler was well connected, charismatic, handsome, charming, and then husband of Annabel Heseltine, daughter of the former deputy Conservative leader Michael Heseltine. Butler had a successful private plastic-surgery practice in addition to his NHS work, and his ambitious and exciting surgical plans made him a media staple. To reporters he was Christiaan Barnard and Dr Kildare rolled into one.

When Butler went public with his face-transplant plans, tabloid journalists harried and pestered surgeons and ethicists, hacking phone lines to track down potential patients. They openly targeted James Partridge, founder of Face Equality International and Changing Faces – whose own face was heavily scarred from burns incurred in a car accident when he was a teenager – publishing an article showing how much 'better' James could look if he had a face transplant.

This media circus perfectly illustrates how our cultural obsession with facial perfection creates impossible pressures. After his car accident, James had spent his entire life championing the rights of visibly different people; he argued repeatedly that society needed to change the way it treated people with visible difference. Until his death in 2020, James was the Chair of my project's Lived Experience Advisory Board. Yet here were newspapers suggesting his face needed 'fixing'.

Understandably, James was furious; he wrote to the then President of the Royal College of Surgeons, Peter Morris (later Sir Peter), to express his concerns that face transplants were being touted as the answer to facial disfigurement, without any evidence, and that potential patients were being harassed.

Sir Peter had a lifelong professional interest in the subject that went beyond being President of the Royal College of Surgeons. His career was in the field of transplantation and immunology. That's why he convened a working party to debate the issue (an unusual act for the Royal College) and brought onto the panel several important surgeons, ethicists and psychologists. Leading advocates and opponents of face transplants were invited to give evidence, including Butler and his friend and patient (and Falklands' War hero), Simon Weston.

Despite the best efforts of the surgical team at the Royal Free, the working party voted against face transplants being carried out in the U.K. – taking the face from a dead donor and laying it over another, living person, seemed at that time too much. Not only because, as medical anthropologists warned, face transplants were potentially replacing one person's identity with another, but also because the immunosuppressant risks were too high.

The Royal College of Surgeons could not prevent any face transplants from going ahead – it was not and is not a regulatory body. But it would be a foolhardy surgeon who went against its judgement; if anything went wrong, and even if it didn't, your professional reputation would be mud.

Inevitably, the Royal Free's efforts collapsed. It must have been a devastating professional and personal blow. Some commentators cited the Royal College's actions as evidence of the U.K.'s backwardness in innovation. Without taking risks, how could the profession advance? To some extent this is true – once the theoretical aspects of a project have been thrashed out, it can only be tested in practice, on the bodies of patients.

But the theoretical aspects were not thrashed out, merely acknowledged. And before any more thought could be had on the matter, the world's first face transplant unexpectedly took place, in another country.

In November 2005 a French team undertook a partial face

transplant on Isabelle Dinoire, a thirty-eight-year-old woman who lived with her daughters and dog, a Labrador cross, in Valenciennes, northern France. Six months earlier, Isabelle had had a disagreement with one of her daughters, who left the house and went to stay overnight with her grandmother. Isabelle, a divorcee, suffered from depression. She took some sleeping tablets and drank alcohol; she was desperate 'to forget', she said. Later there would be disagreement over whether this was a suicide attempt – raising ethical questions about operating on someone who was psychologically vulnerable.

Isabelle fell unconscious. She woke up several hours later, lying on her couch in a pool of blood. Her dog Tania was next to her, 'licking the blood', she said in an interview with *Le Monde*, but it didn't occur to her that it was her blood. Still groggy from the sleeping tablets, Isabelle sat up and tried to light a cigarette but found that it would not stay between her lips. She crawled on hands and knees to the bedroom to look in the mirror. And there she saw a horrific sight. Her dog had chewed away her lips, chin and nose. 'It was not a dream, it was reality. I had no face.'

Isabelle telephoned her mother for help, and since she was barely coherent, her mother called an ambulance. Isabelle spent the next few months in hospital. Almost immediately, her surgeons decided not to undertake standard facial reconstruction; they sent her instead to the Centre Hospitalier Universitaire Amiens-Picardie, 126 kilometres from Valenciennes.

For maxillofacial surgeon Bernard Devauchelle, this was good timing; they had been seeking permission to do a face transplant, and Isabelle was the candidate they had been waiting for. She was grateful to receive such attentive care. Once the paperwork was signed, the waiting game began.

Nobody knew how long it would take for a matching face – one that the bereaved family would be willing to give up – to become available. All that time, Isabelle was waiting in the hospital on standby. Sometimes a helicopter would land outside the hospital and Isabelle would 'wonder, is this the one? Could this be the donor? . . .

when you're waiting for someone to die, to get their face, it's hard to think about these things. But that was the reality.'

In September a call was made to local hospitals to look out for a donor, and by November the family of Maryline St Aubert, who at forty-six had died by suicide, agreed to donate Maryline's face.

In the early hours of 27 November 2005, Devauchelle was working with Jean-Michel Dubernard, the pioneer of hand transplants, whose standing as both surgeon and member of the French National Assembly likely aided in obtaining the ethical permissions. Before Dubernard was brought on board, those permissions, for a more extensive procedure, had been denied.

In a parallel operation, a team of surgeons, led by Sylvie Testelin and Benoît Lengelé, started removing Isabelle's damaged face, peeling away skin, muscle and scar tissue from the area of her nose, mouth and chin, and isolating individual muscles, vessels and nerves.

Isabelle's new face was implanted, and the facial vessels were sutured. There's always an anxious moment when surgeons need to wait to see blood making its way into a transplanted organ: the team was hugely relieved when Isabelle's lips turned pink.

Even at that moment, in the objective and clinical context of the operating theatre, we find gendered ideas about the face and its social meanings.

While Isabelle's female surgeon Sylvie Testelin looked at her patient's new face and wept, feeling the enormous significance of what they had done, her male surgeon Dubernard invited comparisons with Sleeping Beauty, imagining himself as the prince/surgeon who rescued her: 'The donor's face was so beautiful,' he said as he received the prestigious Medawar Prize for his work, 'that I still see her image among the stars in my dreams. When the clamps were released, the colour shot into Isabelle's white lips. This was one of the most moving and magical moments of my life.'

Even in the medical context, we can't escape the fairy-tale narratives about beautiful faces and heroic surgeons that we've encountered throughout this book.

At first, Isabelle made a good recovery, delighting in being able to eat solid food – strawberries, omelettes and chocolate cake. She found she could look in the mirror without horror. And she could leave the hospital without having to wear a surgical mask. While waiting for her operation, she had done this, but because this was France, not Japan or China, masks weren't culturally acceptable, and strangers could be antagonistic.

Later, when Isabelle was famous for having a face transplant, people could still be antagonistic – treating her like 'a circus animal', she said. She was regarded with intrigue and revulsion, like Frankenstein's monster. Her face had been brought back from the grave.

When Isabelle tried to resume a normal life, she found it 'excruciating. I live in a small town and so everyone knew my story . . . Children would laugh at me, and everyone would say, "Look it's her, it's her." [They] would say: "Have you seen her? It's her. It's her . . ." And so, I stopped going out completely.'

Seven years after the face transplant, the scars were still visible, and one of her eyes still drooped. Over time the attention became less 'brutal' and Isabelle more defiant: 'If people stare at me insistently, I don't care any more, I just stare back!'

Public scrutiny was more pronounced because Isabelle was a woman, more judged for her physical appearance than a man would have been. The tabloids obsessed about those lips and asked provocatively whether Isabelle would ever kiss again. They worried about her drinking and smoking, using her mouth for such illicit activities, and they monitored whether she was behaving as an ideal patient.

Isabelle was under constant stress. Her psychological recovery was undermined by the knowledge that at any moment her body might reject her new face. Indeed, in the year after her transplant, this happened twice: her face swelled and turned red, her anti-rejection drugs were adjusted and increased, then the episodes passed.

In 2015, *Le Figaro* magazine reported that Isabelle's body was again rejecting the transplant. And in 2016, Isabelle died from cancer at the age of 49. Her surgeons rejected the possibility that the cancer was connected to her immunosuppressants – which immunologists found strange.

As the working party for the Royal College of Surgeons had feared, Isabelle was never able to adjust to her new face. 'The most difficult thing is to find myself again, as the person I was,' she said, 'with the face I had before the accident, but I know that's not possible.' She acknowledged that she would be for ever attached, physically and emotionally, to her donor, but it was an ambivalent form of gratitude.

Once, Isabelle described how she found a hair on her chin: 'I had never had one. You know it's yours but at the same time "she" is there. I am making her live, but that hair is hers.' Sometimes this sense of inhabiting the same body as another filled her with disgust, as 'having the inside of the mouth of someone else' touching her tongue, 'it was atrocious'. And yet Isabelle also felt appreciation: 'When I look in the mirror, I see a mixture of the two [of us]. The donor is always with me. She saved my life.'

If our face is who we are, what happens when we wear someone else's? Isabelle's experience suggests that identity doesn't simply transfer with the physical tissue – instead, you live with a strange sense of hosting another person's presence. Robert Chelsea said the same thing to me – that when he looks in the mirror, he sees himself, and his donor.

Robert has never found out who his donor was, though he has written via the hospital to the family, expressing his interest in meeting. Isabelle knew who her donor was. After the name was leaked by a British tabloid, she searched the internet for information about Maryline and said that she wanted to meet her family, to thank them for their 'magical donation'. When newspapers broke the story that Maryline had died by hanging, Isabelle reported feeling a kind of sisterhood with the dead woman that was stronger than life. This was a woman who had suffered as Isabelle had, who had died by suicide, which Isabelle was said to have attempted, and now the women were forever united in a single face.

Isabelle's experience suggests that the Royal College of Surgeons was right to be cautious, that there was much uncertainty about the psychological impact of receiving another person's face. Isabelle was not resilient enough, her surgeons decided, acknowledging that she was not an 'ideal patient'. But who would be, in such circumstances? Isabelle was also never offered traditional reconstructive surgery – and how can a real choice be made without all options being available? She was encouraged to sign a publicity agreement, which meant she would profit from the media sale of photographs and a subsequent film. She later participated in a book about her journey, entitled *Isabelle's Kiss*.

These ethical complexities were not debated; the surgical proof had been made. Any reservations about identity fell by the wayside and the face race began – with face transplants taking place in China, the U.S., Turkey, Spain, Italy.

Few people know that Isabelle's transplant ultimately failed; that though her operation was heralded as a new dawn in transplantation, her transplanted lips became necrotic and had to be removed. She asked her surgeons to replace her transplant with a graft from her own body, because she could not bear to be buried without her face. There was far less media attention surrounding her death in 2016 than had accompanied her transplant.

There are echoes here of heart transplantation. The first 'successful' heart transplant patient, Louis Washansky, a South African aged fifty-four, lived only eighteen days afterwards in 1967 – just long enough to meet the press, have his photo taken – and ensure the subsequent global fame of his surgeon, Christiaan Barnard. Human heart transplants are now so routine that surgeons are experimenting with xenotransplantation, transplanting cells or organs from one species to another, for example using pig hearts. But hearts are essential to life. And face transplants are not.

Leaving aside the medical challenges, the success of a face transplant cannot be evaluated as a purely surgical act, as if achieved in a vacuum. Any meaningful measurement needs to consider how the transplant affects a person's body and their world: their health, work, living arrangements, friendships, family support, state of mind. When evaluating patients for face transplants, too many surgeons tend to be more concerned with what is surgically possible, and with the short term. They might evaluate a patient's social support networks before surgery, but not afterwards, when that support often falls away.

Race matters as well as gender in face transplants. Robert Chelsea had to wait a lot longer than Isabelle Dinoire for a new face. There are far fewer African American organ and blood donors than among white people, and for good reason. During slavery, Black people were routinely experimented on without anaesthetic – Dr J. Marion Sims's gynaecological experiments in the nineteenth century are a case in point – in the grotesque belief that Black people were closer to animals and did not feel pain. That beliefs about race impacted how faces were viewed was shown in chapter two; Black faces did not conjure the same sympathy or emotional engagement, because Black people were routinely compared to brute animals or mocked as minstrels.

Between the 1930s and the 1970s there were repeated scandals about race and medicine, such as the infamous Tuskegee Syphilis Study in Alabama. In a medical experiment funded by the U.S. Public Health Service, researchers recruited 600 Black men, 399 with untreated syphilis and 201 without the disease. The men were told they were receiving free healthcare for 'bad blood', without any explanation what that meant; those who had syphilis were never told and their informed consent was not sought. Treatment was deliberately withheld, even after penicillin was discovered as a cure. Many participants died, went blind, infected their wives and children, developed horrific facial wounds, or died.

Black and Hispanic patients continue to be affected by healthcare disparities in the U.S. Inevitably, given this history, there remains distrust in medical systems, and racism is still built into healthcare structures.

During his pre-transplant evaluation, Robert Chelsea tells me, it was presumed he didn't have a supportive family network, because of a stereotype – that Black men are feckless and desert their families. The forms used for his psychological evaluation were based on generalizations from white communities – the presumption that he might have been suicidal, for instance, appalled Robert (suicide is far more common among white people). And the first face he was offered was noticeably paler than his own.

At the beginning, the hospital offered Robert a choice of four colour options for his donor face. This might work for white skin, but it simply doesn't for Black skin tones, where there is far more colour diversity. After Robert turned down the first donor face he was offered, the hospital learned from their experience and extended the range of skin tones to eighteen possible shades. Robert felt comfortable receiving a donor face with any shade between eight and sixteen on the scale, and later, when there weren't enough donors to secure a match, he reduced the lightest acceptable tone to number five.

Robert knew that a lighter face would mean he would be treated differently, that he would self-identify differently too. Even though our faces are 'ours', we 'see' ourselves in the faces of our families, it helps us to know our history, it affirms our identity and sense of belonging. As we saw in our discussions of photography and historical facial reconstruction, that sense of visual history matters, personally, nationally, and even as a species.

We can see the desire to be part of one's ancestry in the case of Katie Stubblefield, the young white girl whose story of attempted suicide and subsequent face transplant were published in *National Geographic* magazine (earning Maggie Steber and Lynn Johnson a well-deserved Pulitzer Prize nomination).

In 2014, Katie, a beautiful eighteen-year-old living with her family in Mississippi, became distressed when she found text messages to another girl on her boyfriend's phone. She placed the barrel of her brother's .308-calibre hunting rifle beneath her chin and pointed upwards, before pulling the trigger. Katie narrowly missed death, but she lost most of her face, including her sight;

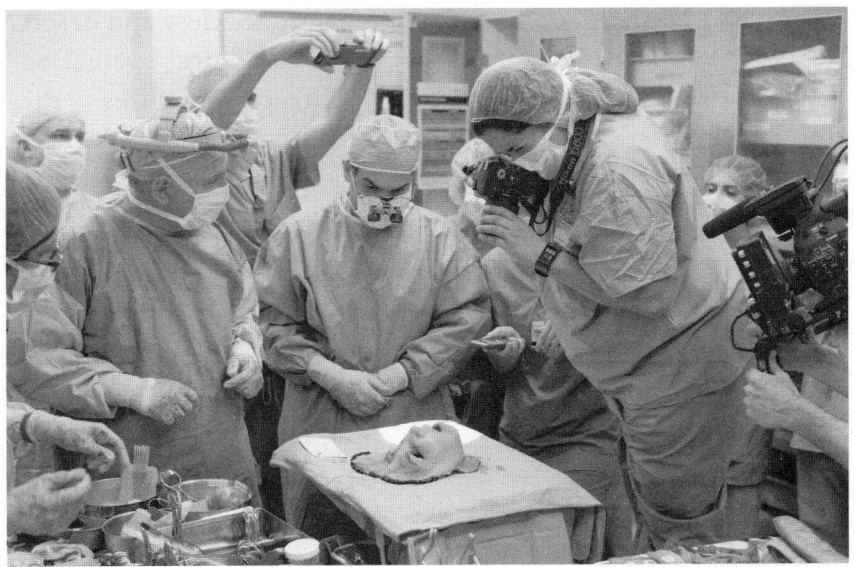

36. Lynn Johnson, Katie Stubblefield's new face, before transplant, 2017.

her brain was exposed. Three years later, after multiple life-saving surgeries, Katie became the youngest person ever to undergo a face transplant (fig. 36).

But the transplant itself was not straightforward. Katie's parents were in the waiting room throughout their daughter's surgery. Part of the way through, her surgeons came out of theatre – they had hit a snag. There was an unintended mismatch between the donor face and Katie's skull, and the face looked too large for the operation as it had been planned.

Would the parents prefer for Katie to receive a triangle that included the nose, mouth and chin, which would have a poorer aesthetic outcome, or for her to receive the whole face?

Among all the unthinkable decisions that Katie's parents had to make, this one must have been particularly difficult – and they didn't agree. Katie's father wanted his daughter to have the entire face transplant so that she looked as attractive as possible. But Katie's mother wanted a partial transplant – so that they could minimize the risks. In the end, Katie received the whole face. In photographs released by the hospital and published in *National Geographic*, the new face was much larger than her tiny frame.

Yet when Katie's mother looked at her daughter's face after the transplant, she saw a family likeness – it was her mother's nose, she said. The donor's grandmother said the same thing; she saw her granddaughter's nose – their family inheritance. How often do we see what we want to see in the face? Perhaps we are no more objective than the creators of Victorian dioramas.

In all of this, the donor family has been overlooked. Even the Royal College of Surgeons didn't think about the emotional effects on families, beyond the concern that a recipient might look like the donor. What resemblance there is will come from skin tone, colour and texture, and the same nose – which, being cartilaginous and bony only at the top, will keep its own shape. Facial hair, too, will grow in the same way as it did on the donor face. Even without an exact match, then, there's enough of the original face for the donor family to relate to.

This challenge is made more complex by the language of organ donation. It is expected to be a selfless act from the donor to the recipient; it's also often framed as a way for the family of the donor to achieve closure. Recipients are expected and assumed to feel grateful for the 'gift' they receive from strangers. This kind of language introduces a sense of emotional entanglement – I've spoken to many recipients who describe themselves as 'not good enough' for the organs they have received, and who worry that a sacrifice has been made in vain.

Which forces a question: Is a gift still a gift if it belongs, even in some emotional or symbolic way, to the donor and their family?

Robert Chelsea is keen to meet his donor family, but considerate enough to be aware that they might not want to meet him. And he worries that the physical disparity between himself and their loved one might not be well received. They might not like the way it fits, 'because the shape of my head is different, my frame is smaller'.

Not all recipient and donor family members are given choices about when and how to meet. When Ebony first saw her father after his transplant, she was not able to do so in the privacy of the hospital. Instead, the hospital media office arranged for her to meet Robert at home, where the television cameras were waiting.

This raises some red flags. It does not safeguard the well-being of Ebony or her father, or their relationship. But it's a common theme in accounts of face transplants in the U.S., where some hospitals do not show appropriate regard for the non-surgical impacts on patients, their families and the donor families. Promotion of a face transplant wins grants and allows clinics to advertise – which brings them an important income stream.

In 2008, Connie Culp received the first face transplant in the U.S., in an operation performed by Maria Siemionow. Connie later appeared on *Oprah* and ABC news, where she met Becky, the daughter of her donor Anna Kasper. The meeting took place on camera, and in the moments before it took place Becky was visibly distressed – 'I just really wanna hug her,' she said. When she saw Connie, Becky noticed that she had her mother's 'perfect nose'. Becky did hug Connie – and seemed emotionally overwhelmed.

When Cameron Underwood turned up for his face transplant, following a suicide attempt, he was introduced by his surgeon Eduardo Rodriguez to the mother of his donor, who was still on life support. How could Cameron have turned down a meeting with that tearful mother; how could Cameron's mother have resisted a hug from the woman who thanked her for letting her own son 'live on'?

We can't always know what people are feeling in such situations, but we can see the emotional reactions and wonder how we might respond. When another of Rodriguez's patients, the firefighter Patrick Hardison, received a face transplant from a young cyclist, David Rodebaugh, Patrick was introduced to David's mother, Nancy Millar. News cameras watched as Nancy stared at and hugged Patrick. She said she wanted to kiss Patrick's forehead, in the same place she'd always kissed it during the twenty-six years when that face had belonged to her son.

Surely, we cannot use the same language of a 'gift' or 'giving' for face transplants that we use for other, less visible and emotionally affecting organs. In these cases, the face feels more like a loan.

There are also other unresolved ethical challenges. Most leaders of face-transplant teams in American hospitals are plastic surgeons, many of whom have their own private practice. As hospitals win major grants on the back of these operations, so plastic surgeons can use their face-transplant expertise to drum up private clients for cosmetic surgery, advertising their services on social media. To date, there's no regulation of this.

By contrast, face-transplant recipients in the U.S. tend not to be wealthy. They set up GoFundMe campaigns, for example, to support themselves financially, or to raise funds for the transplant. Patients who have received face transplants are usually unable to find work afterwards, and are without long-term financial support. Many can't afford to pay for rent, medication and travelling to specialized hospitals. On top of that, they need to deal with extended wait times for treatment, surgeons who are hard to get hold of, and, ultimately, systemic issues such as kidney failure or cancer due to their use of immunosuppressant drugs. Face transplants affect the whole body, not just the face.

These economic realities reveal something crucial about how face transplants work. We like to imagine medicine as being above commercial concerns, but face transplants exist in a world where surgeons become celebrities, hospitals compete for prestige and patients struggle to afford basic care. It's the same commodification of faces we've seen throughout this book, taken to its logical extreme.

And what of the effects on team members? Plastic surgeons often consider themselves artists, as we saw when discussing cosmetic surgery. But many actual artists work in hospitals, and they do not consider the face to be just an organ. During the hundreds of interviews that I conducted with hospital staff and patients internationally, I met a prosthetist: someone who makes prosthetics to replace parts of the face – noses, eyes, ears, cheeks – the patient has lost. I'll call her Sarah. Sarah did not feel aligned with the multidisciplinary face-transplant team with which she worked.

When I visited her, we sat surrounded by fragments of faces: a plaster cast of a nose sat on Sarah's desk; a glass eye and a silicone cheek on her shelf; an upturned plastic mould was sitting on a stack of photocopying paper, as though left there when she moved from one task to another. Sarah is young; early thirties maybe, with large brown eyes beneath a heavy fringe, and she was recently involved in a face-transplant procedure where she was required to make a replica of the donor's face for burial.

Creating a replacement donor face is common in face transplants – partly for cultural reasons, so that bodies can be viewed if desired, partly to keep up the narrative of caring for the dead body, and partly to respect the feelings of hospital and mortuary attendants. These replicas are traditionally made from silicone and are often 3D printed. It was not part of Sarah's job when she first came to the clinic, where she worked mostly with patients who needed replacement noses or eyes. I asked her how she felt about making a face for the donor. Her gaze dropped to the floor, and she replied: 'It's difficult. I like my job. I understand that it needs to be done. But the face – it's so personal.'

Surgeons and prosthetists alike deal with bodies that are suffering and in need of care, but the relationships that they have with those bodies are necessarily different. Surgeons can be notoriously poor communicators. And most of the time that matters less than that they know exactly what to do with a scalpel and an open body. Sarah told me how much she liked the face-transplant team personally; they were good guys. (And most were guys. Very few women become face-transplant surgeons, like Maria Siemionow; only 12 per cent of transplant surgeons are female. As a rule, women plastic surgeons work in reconstructive rather than cosmetic surgery, though there is overlap.)

These guys might laugh and joke with colleagues, Sarah said, but they would also spend hours hunched over a cadaver, teasing apart the nerves, the fibres and the vessels of a face that's about to be transplanted. The time spent on cadavers is a rehearsal, too, for the hours the transplant surgery itself would involve. When Cameron Underwood received a new face from Eduardo Rodriguez's team in New York, more than one hundred people worked for twenty-five hours on the transplant, which included the upper and lower jaw, the nose, and all thirty-two teeth along with gums, lower eyelids, and parts of the cheek and forehead.

The last body that Sarah had worked on belonged to a thirty-one-year-old man, whom we will call Mike. He was white, smooth-skinned, engaged to be married. He had a small tattoo of a salamander on his left forearm. On his way home from work one day a car had pulled out from a junction, T-boning his motorcycle and sending him over its handlebars. He had landed on his head, breaking his neck instantly. Now he lay still and motionless but alive, alone as his family had said their goodbyes, knowing that the organ-retrieval team would soon arrive, to do their work before the life support was switched off. Mike had always been an organ donor, had wanted in life to give others a 'second chance'. His distraught family had found some comfort in that, a hope to cling to as they imagined the bodies and families that might benefit.

When the transplant liaison team asked about Mike's organs, the family had agreed in an instant to donate. Everything that was useful they could take. Yes, even his face. That was the kind of guy Mike was – he wanted to help anyone he could. When this message was relayed to Sarah, she wanted to make the most beautiful image of Mike's face that she could, even if his family would never see it.

Before the organ-retrieval teams arrived, Sarah took a plaster cast of Mike's face from which to create his mask. She found Mike stripped naked beneath a white hospital sheet, his body still attached to life support, with a tracheotomy that kept his lungs filling with oxygen, his chest moving up and down. Mike's brain was medically dead, but because his heart was beating, an essential measure to keep the organs alive and perfused with blood, his skin was still warm.

Sarah perched on the edge of his bed and arranged her equipment, then applied an alginate impression material to his face and waited for it to set. She would use the mould she was creating to make an exact silicone replica of Mike's face; she would match it to his skin tone and add any identifying marks – the mole above his right eye, the freckles on his nose, a chickenpox scar on his chin – from photographs his family had supplied.

When the mould was ready to be removed, Sarah peeled it away and cleaned Mike's face. She tucked his sheet back beneath his shoulders, and took the plaster cast back to her office, where she set to work. When the organ-procurement team had arrived, and taken not only Mike's organs that would save other lives, but his face too, it was her job to return to Mike's body and lay her handiwork over the naked gap where his face – the warm face she had modelled, and touched and washed – used to be.

To my knowledge, no family of a face-transplant donor has asked to see the body after the face has been removed. But the fact that using a mask in this way remains an important stage in the donation process highlights the face's enduring emotional importance, even in medical contexts.

Would Mike still have been Mike, once his own face was removed, before the replica was attached? This is a complex philosophical and legal question. If we think about identity as being tied to appearance, especially the face in the age of facehood, then does altering it change who we are?

Who we are is surely more about our mind, our consciousness, beliefs and personality rather than our appearance. Yet the fact that we would not ask the same question if Mike's leg or arm or kidney were removed shows the unique status of the face in popular understandings of identity.

Legally we do not need a face to be a recognized human being, but according to the French philosopher Emmanuel Levinas, seeing the face of another obliges us to acknowledge their humanity and respond to them ethically. We have seen throughout this book that the face plays a strong symbolic role in how society and individuals perceive personhood and generate empathy and compassion.

But Levinas's argument did not include the experiences of people with disabilities, including visual impairment. Are blind people not included in the world of the human because they cannot see faces? What of the ways we encounter others through the other senses – touch, sound, or speech? And historically, societies haven't treated other humans (let alone animals) ethically just because they have faces – which suggests that some faces matter more than others in practice.

All of us experience facial changes during our lifetimes. But to lose a face through accident or disease, rather than mere ageing, propels people like Isabelle and Robert and Katie, and all face-transplant recipients, into a difficult new world – one often linked to loss of sight, of ease, of opportunities, and even of autonomy.

We don't know how far a face transplant affects people's sense of self, because we don't yet know what questions to ask. We've seen that donor families are neglected too; we don't know how they feel about the continued survival of their loved ones' faces, though many families of face-transplant patients have thanked donor families for letting their kin 'live on'. We don't know how those families feel when the faces, and the recipients, die. Could it be a second bereavement? And we don't know how recipients' families feel, because they haven't been asked either. Some family members, though, such as Robert Chelsea's daughter Ebony, have been vocal about their discomfort. She doesn't look at her father in the same way now. 'I only know it's him when he opens his mouth,' she says.

The face, in the end, is both everything and nothing. It's the first thing we notice about each other and the last thing that truly matters about who we are. Face transplants force us to confront this paradox directly. In trying to give people new faces, we discover that the face we seek – the one that will make us whole, acceptable, loveable – might not exist at all. It might be that what we're really seeking is not a new face, but a new world: one that doesn't judge us so harshly for the faces we already have.

Afterword

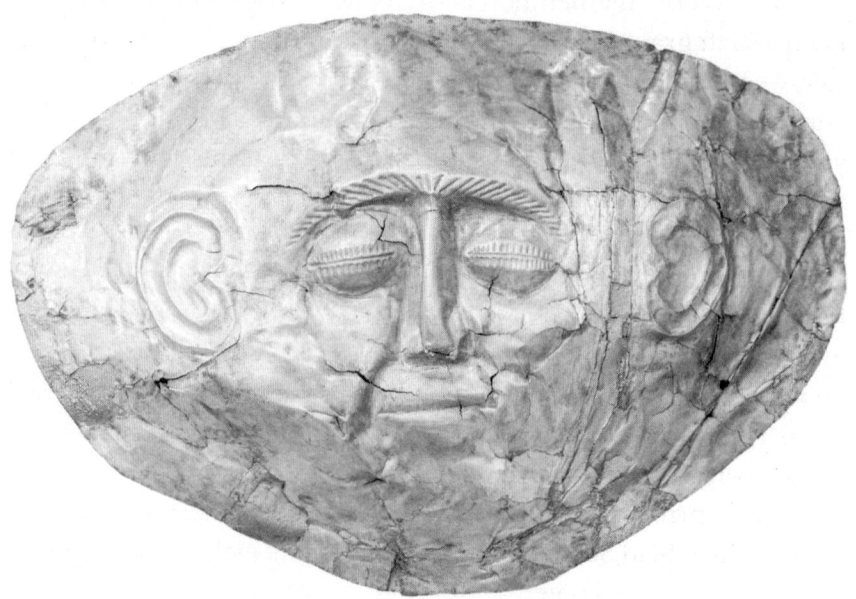

37. Unknown artist, Mask of Agamemnon, c. 1500 BCE.

There is no getting away from the human face – from birth to death, it defines us. It does so even before birth and after death, as we saw in foetal scanning, and the death mask – the *imago* (image) used in ancient Rome. There is much more to say about both these themes, but no book can be exhaustive, especially one on the human face. So, I will conclude by journeying back to the Mycenaean civilization we encountered in the chapter on portraiture, and a story that brings together many of the threads raised in this book, about appearance and reality, authenticity and trickery, the individual and the social face. Meet the Mask of Agamemnon (fig. 37).

In 1876 the German archaeologist Heinrich Schliemann was

excavating at Mycenae, the site of a major centre of ancient Greek civilization. He was searching for the Tomb of Agamemnon, the legendary king of Mycenae, and leader of the Greek army in the Trojan War, as described in Homer's *Iliad*. When the excavations revealed five shaft graves inside the citadel walls filled with treasures, Schliemann believed his quest had been successful.

The Mask of Agamemnon is one of several gold masks retrieved from a shaft grave, masks that had been buried with the dead alongside weapons and other valuables. The mask was with a body that was dressed in a breastplate, including an armlet and a necklace, and surrounded by weapons and two silver vases. Many weapons were also heaped on top of the body, indicating high status and prestige. The mask was not an actual death mask, but hammered out from a gold sheet, and designed to resemble a human face; it has stylized features such as almond-shaped eyes, a moustache and a beard. Schliemann believed the mask had a Greek physiognomy and profile, and that it could only have belonged to the mythical king. 'I have gazed upon the face of Agamemnon,' he allegedly told King George of Greece in a telegram.

Some controversy followed over whether that mask was authentic, or a fake. Had Schliemann orchestrated an elaborate hoax?

We can see why contemporaries were suspicious – by linking the mask's discovery to the Homeric legend, Schliemann could seal his fame and fulfil the Victorian desire to date European lineage back to the Greeks that we saw in the chapter on reconstructed faces. At a time of great academic and public interest in History, there were several contemporary archaeological hoaxes, most famously the Calaveras skull found in California (1866) and, later, the Piltdown Man in Sussex (1912), both of which toyed with the story of human evolution.

Most scholars today believe that the mask was found in the grave rather than being planted, but also, that it never belonged to Agamemnon. The mask has been dated to a much earlier time, 1550–1500 BCE, several centuries before the Trojan War supposedly took place. Given its economic value, the mask probably did belong to a Mycenaean noble or ruler, but we do not know who that was.

The authenticity of the mask mattered a great deal to Schliemann, who wanted to prove that Homer's epic poems were based on real events. But it didn't matter to national pride – the Mask of Agamemnon is still called that and housed in the National Archaeological Museum of Athens as part of a grand narrative of the Bronze Age. And it need not matter to us; the existence of the mask shows the symbolic importance of the face as a figurehead, and Schliemann's quest illustrates our search to find some emotional, personal or national inheritance in the human face.

Many such funeral masks have been made throughout history, most memorably the funeral masks used in Ancient Egypt, such as the Mask of Tutankhamun. Death masks were more realistic, since they were moulded from the face of a dead person, and their main function from the fourteenth century CE was to help sculptors create realistic statues and busts; from the 1800s such death masks became artistic and commemorative objects, given emotional meaning (sometimes even relic status) through their literal contact with a person, as well as their physical resemblance.

Masks have been made to honour, and mock, people, but also to 'save face', literally and symbolically. The English word 'mask' first appeared in the 1530s, from the Middle French *masque*, meaning a covering to guard the face. The Greek language is more expansive, and it recognizes the different meanings that masks can have – *prosopon* means 'face', 'mask', 'appearance' and 'manifestation'. *Persona* was the Greek term used for a strategic mask that is worn in public, to show the social role that one adopts.

Masks can hide as well as reveal our emotions. We expect to see evidence of a person's emotions on their face – at least in Western cultures; in expressions of empathy and pity, we respond to the emotional need conveyed by tears or sorrow. And this makes us responsible towards one another, as the philosopher Emmanuel Levinas observed; we cannot help but see ourselves, and our common humanity, in the faces of others.

Yet there is always an element of performance to our emotional expressions, and in what we reveal; consciously or otherwise, we curate and manage our faces to make them socially acceptable. In ancient Greek theatre, actors made this link between emotions and performance literal by wearing masks to signify the character they were playing, and to convey distinct emotions like joy, sadness, or anger. In Japanese theatre from the fourteenth century, the classical drama of *noh* similarly uses masks to convey character and feeling – *noh* traditionally employed 60 basic types; today over 200 are in use. Some of those emotions are not acceptable to show in real life; we have seen that Japanese culture is traditionally more restrained in terms of emotional display than their Western counterparts, and less dedicated to the cult of the individual.

In all these ways, in identifying a person, in communicating and hiding emotions, and in the display codes that make us human, the face takes centre stage.

And yet, the face is a paradox – it is both the essence of our individual identity and the thing that gives us facehood, but it also fundamentally conveys a social message. Its meaning is only fully realized in and through our relationships – without the ability to communicate with others, in expressions, in speech, in sensation, the face is just a mask.

Think about everything we've explored in this book. Remember how portrait painters first made faces into markers of individual identity. How photographers turned everyone into a potential subject, making faces democratic but also vulnerable to surveillance. How cosmetic surgeons promised to perfect faces, and recognition technology learned to track them. How face transplants literally turned faces into commodities that could be removed, transported and installed on someone else.

Each of these developments contributed to, and ultimately challenged, the notion of facehood, the assertion that we are individually and uniquely reducible to our faces. And our faces are layered, throughout our lives, with racialized, gendered presumptions, before we open our eyes, let alone our mouths.

It is difficult to let go of these belief systems; they are encoded into our culture, our imagination, our thoughts, and perhaps even our genes. We have inherited and reproduced myths of beauty and goodness (and ugliness and evil) since the classical period, and today they benefit consumer conglomerates – why would we buy so much to enhance our face, and do so much to improve our looks, if we didn't believe it would make us happier, sexier, younger, healthier, more successful, and even more loved? And if it does not? Well, we must not be doing it right.

What about the other claims made about the face, such as, that we know what people are thinking and feeling because their face betrays them? Sometimes, perhaps, but that's not the only way – and what about the social masks and systems that hide the ways we really feel? What about cultural differences and mixed feelings and ambivalence? Or the ways we project onto others traits and characters that are stereotypical rather than deserved?

None of us is immune to these delusions – we inherit, internalize and reproduce them; it's how systemic racism and patriarchy make their way beneath the skin. We could be more conscious, though, when it happens, and more thoughtful about why. Otherwise, we will simply invest future faces with the lazy shorthand of the past.

Take social robots – we might worry about whether robots might become sentient, Terminator-style, but we overlook how they reinforce traditional gender hierarchies. Most robots and virtual assistants are created female, especially service robots that deal with conventionally female activities such as care and domesticity; most sex robots are also female. Making service robots female and passive increases the tendency for live women to be regarded in those terms too.

Not all social robots have faces, but most female humanoid robots or 'gynoids' are white skinned, with pronounced breasts, soft voices and demure facial expressions. Sophia was modelled on the Hollywood actress Audrey Hepburn, and has long brown hair, white teeth and smooth skin. On the American programme *The Tonight Show* she was wheeled out by her male creator to flirt with Jimmy Fallon, who acted as though it was a typical first date, only to be 'creeped out' by how real she seemed.

This connects directly to what we saw in our exploration of cosmetic surgery and beauty ideals – the same narrow standards of attractiveness that drive people to surgical enhancement are now literally built into our artificial companions. The robots reflect our own cultural biases about what faces should look like.

Most robots are not just modelled after white celebrities but also made from shiny white material. Why does that matter? Well, a study conducted by the Human Interface Technology Laboratory in New Zealand – Robots and Racism – suggests this subtle colour coding taps into our subconscious imaginings about race. We give robots a race too, and attribute racial stereotypes to them. In one shooter test, images of Black and White people and robots were flashed onto a screen and people told to 'shoot' those holding a weapon. Black robots not holding weapons were shot more often than white ones.

We have seen all this before, and not just with Google Images inadvertently labelling Black faces as 'gorillas' due to biased algorithms. When a Taiwanese American woman, Joz Wang, bought a Nikon Coolpix camera in 2009 she found it couldn't read the faces of her family; each time a person smiled, the camera popped up an error message: 'DID SOMEONE BLINK?' And Microsoft's Xbox Kinect had a controller that used facial and bodily movement to control a video game; that controller repeatedly failed to recognize players with darker skin. As they say in machine learning, garbage in, garbage out; a technology is only as good as its data.

Real-looking faces are hard to reproduce, robotics engineers tell me, especially around the eyes and mouths, where humans are most expressive. Artists, too, fret about the eyes because they are so important to capture character; my friend Eleanor Crook tells me that there's always a moment, when she's modelling a face in clay, when its eyes seem suddenly to come to life – and that's when she knows her work is done.

Of course, human faces are even more complex and difficult to get right – not only because the tissue around the eyes is thin and delicate and, like the mouth, highly mobile – but also because both areas have intricate networks of muscles, nerves and blood vessels. And aside from these flesh-and-blood considerations, there are all those other components to consider, cultural, emotional and communicative.

We forget about the craft involved in the creation of a real face, because we are used to thinking of it as natural, rather than a work of art, an artefact, in the traditional sense of the word, that is, 'an object made or modified by human workmanship'.

This book has shown that the face is just as much an artefact as the Mask of Agamemnon – crafted, shaped and displayed in ways that are both personal and a product of history. From the moment portrait painters learned to capture individual identity, through photography's democratization of faces, to cosmetic surgery's promise of perfection, and recognition technology's surveillance of our every expression, we have been actively constructing what faces mean.

Now what do we do with this knowledge? How do we live with faces in a world that both obsesses over them and fundamentally misunderstands them?

Perhaps we start by questioning the very premise of facehood – the idea that our faces are who we are. Perhaps we resist the pressure to perfect our faces through surgery, filters, or any other technological intervention, and instead work to create a world that values human worth beyond appearance. Perhaps we demand that the technologies being built today – from social robots to recognition systems – reflect the full diversity of human faces rather than perpetuating narrow, biased ideals.

Because how we choose to craft our faces, shape their meaning, and display them in the future, is still up for grabs. The question is whether we'll continue to let commercial interests, ancient prejudices and technological biases define what faces mean – or whether we will resist.

Anything is possible. The face, after all, is not just our individual inheritance. It's our collective creation. And like any artefact, it can be reimagined, reshaped and remade. The only question is: how do we want to face the future?

Index

Actisanes (Ethiopian king), founder of Rhinocorura, 8
Adler, Alfred, and the inferiority complex, 101
Adomakoh-Young, Isabel, actor and drag king, 87
advertising: origins and value, 83; credulity 92; defining success, 94; photography, 99; ubiquity, 112; emotional responses (AI), 153; ubiquity of faces, 200; cosmetic surgery 232
Aegean art, 4–5
ageing: Roman sculptural portraits, 9; self-consciousness, 93; cosmetic surgery, 111, 113; 'resting bitch face', 157; dementia, 206
Albert, Prince, on his death bed, 46
Alexander the Great: coinage, 10–11; birth mythology, 115
Alexandria, anatomy school, 5–6
algorithms: facial recognition technology, 63; beauty, 106–9; detecting foetal alcohol syndrome, 133; misplaced trust in, 153; racism, 159
American Society of Plastic Surgeons: childhood bullying, 103; cosmetic surgery, 108
amygdala: emotions, 152; as 'fear' centre, 190
anatomical dissection: classical, 5–6; Renaissance, 14; Burke and Hare, 14–15, 118; Vesalius and Leonardo, 142; forensic facial reconstruction, 163
anatomy: function and senses, xxi; knowledge, 5; Renaissance, 14, 23; and expression, 139; CT scanning, 168; brain, 197
anchor bias: evolutionary science, 105; modern evolutionary psychology 178
anger, *see also* expression: medieval, 16; Le Brun's *Method*, 25, 144; humours, 59–60; Charles Darwin, 84; experiments, 146; teeth baring, 148; one of six basic emotions, 152; gender, 156; racism, 158; as cultural construct, 155–6
animal faces: cave art, 3; physiognomy, 7–8; consciousness, 84; self-recognition, 85–6, 204–5; expressions, 138; vivisection, 139, 142; Darwin's *Expressions of Emotions*, 146; autism and communication, 199; same-species recognition, 205; racist comparisons, 227
anonymity: and urbanization, 15; Munch's *Scream*, 32; fear of crime, 48; Victorian identity concerns, 51; of photographic medical subjects, 149; goal of face transplant, 214
ants: identity and recognition, 205

Index

anthropology: criminal, 32; Victorian, 48; comparative physiognomy, 60; geographical comparison, 73; photography, 83; Boas and ethnocentrism, 150; Mead and cultural variation, 151; history of emotion, 154; Artificial Intelligence, 159; forensic facial reconstruction, 160, 164–5; palaeoanthropology, 166–7; forensic anthropology, 168; Neanderthals, 181; medical anthropology, 221

archaeology: cave art, 3; anthropology, 160; Neanderthals, 165, 177–9, 238; forensic facial reconstruction, 168

architecture: Greek, 5; golden ratio, 6; Christian architecture, 11; interior design and mirrors, 76–7

Aristotle: physiognomy, 6–11; Victorian science, 42, 49, 56–8; St Jerome, 140; classification of emotions, 142

artists: early human, 3–4; Cubist, 5; Medieval, 15–16; Renaissance, 14, 142; symbolism, 16; emotions, 18; enhanced status of, 19, 144; cost of painted portraits, 22–3; reusing faces, 24; the science of painting, 25, 143; slave labour, 27; patronage, 29–30; photography, 32; modern art, 33; experimentation, 35; photographic artists, 40; camera obscura use, 43; humanism and classical values, 69; emotions, 70, 145; mirrors, 74, 80; the art of surgery, 109; performance art, 111; forensic and paleo artists, 163–4, 170–73, 243; art and science, 179–81; prosthetists, 232–3

autism, *see also* neurodivergence: expressions, 156–7; prosopagnosia, 193; brain scans, 198; pareidolia, 199

Azure Face (emotion-recognition software), 153, 159

babies, *see also* foetuses: Renaissance painting, 115–16; maternal influence, 121; impact of birth on faces, 130–131; 'face hunger', 191; 'Baby Face Model', 134; healthcare inequalities, 132, 134; Other Race Effect, 132; 'baby schema', 136; smell, 186; recognizing caregivers, 187

Bacon, Francis (twentieth-century artist), 1, 32–3; *Study after Velázquez's Portrait of Pope Innocent X*, 34–5

Bacon, Francis (philosopher), 143

Baroque style, 30–31

Barrett, Lisa Feldman, and the emotional brain, 154–6

beards: Jesus Christ, 18; measurement of, 56; Lombroso's criminals, 59; shaving, 77; forensic facial reconstruction, 170; Greek profile, 239; on transplanted faces, 230

beauty: morality, xix, 36; the golden ratio, 6, 106–7; spirituality, 8; gender and idealization, 10, 30; lightness, 42; Egyptian grooming, 71; 'mouches', 79; cosmetics and display, 81; and whiteness, 82; fashion, 83; beauty standards, shift in, 91, 102; tutorials, 93; correlation with success, 94; in cinema, 99; cosmetic

Index

surgery and consumerism, 89, 101; patriarchy, 104; Victorian bias, 105; algorithms, 106, 109; Eurocentrism, 105–7, 110, 203; racism, 108; Nazis, 108; ORLAN, 111, robot faces, 243

before-and-after, *see also* fairy stories, 92–6; 218

Bell, Sir Charles, 146

Berger, John, *Ways of Seeing*, 91

Bertillon, Alphonse, 56–8

biometrics: the unique face, xviii; non-visual indicators, 86; gait, 53, 77, 189, 192, 205; Victorian measurement, 54; Bertillonage, 56–60; face as data, 61, 63; counterterrorism, 64; scent, 186; and prosopagnosia, 205

Blackface, *see also* racism, 108

Black portraiture: European servants, 26–8; Juan de Pareja, 27; Olaudah Equiano, 28; caricatures, 182; Black-owned photographic studios, 60; Frederick Douglass, 60

Bodamer, Joachim, and acquired prosopagnosia, 184, 187, 190, 204

Body Dysmorphia Disorder (BDD), *see also* mental health, 89

Bogart, Kathleen, 137–8

Botox: and facial expression, 139–40; unregulated, 95, 97, 104–5, 114, emotions, 139, 177

Botticelli, Alessandro, *Birth of Venus*, 1

Boucher, François, 30; *Pompadour at her Toilette* (1750), 81

Broca, Paul, 165, 190

Brontë, Emily, *Wuthering Heights* (1847), 31–2, 58

brows: furrowed, 9; in anger, 25; and ageing, 156; emotions, 31–2; measuring, 49, 58; receding in criminals, 59; grooming, 77, 79; co-evolution in dogs, 86; gender, 87, 104; glabella, 90; fashion, 102; in micro-expressions, 139; the third eye, 145; in Neanderthals, 167, 178; Adrien Brody, 203

bulls, *see also* animal faces, in cave painting, 3

bureaucracy: distinguishing people, 11, classifying people, 42; physiognomy, 49; social order, 50; colonial, 53; biometrics, 54; passports, 62

Burke, William, 14, 118

Burton, Mike, 191–3, 200–1

Butler, Peter, 220, 221

Cadaval, Duchesse de, toilette set of, 80

camera obscura, 38, 43, 67, 70

Caravaggio, 30, 69–70; *Narcissus at the Fountain*, 69

caricatures: and racism, 55, Black people and Jews, 108, 182; emotions, 144

Carroll, Lewis, *Through the Looking Glass*, 67

cartes de visite, 45–7, 62

cave art: meanings, xxii, Chauvet-Pont-d'Arc and Lascaux valley, 3–4; public interest in, 166

Charlemagne, Roman emperor, 14

Chaucer, Geoffrey, *The Canterbury Tales*, 15

cheekbones: Lombroso's criminals, 59; cosmetic surgery, 92; gender affirmation, 104; leading men, 202–3

Chelsea, Robert, 208–10, 212–17, 225–8, 230–31, 236

Index

children: drawing faces, 1; Roman portraiture, 10; using mirrors, 73, 86, 154; Freud and Darwin, 83–4; bullied for appearance, 103; medical diagnoses, 134; caring for children, 136; 'Ginx's Baby', 147; and primates, 148; prosopagnosia, 192, 195, 198–199, 205

chins: 'Zoom chin', xxv; strength, 11; determined, 20; measured by Galton, 58; weak chins of criminals, 59; cosmetic surgery, 105; Botticelli's *Venus* and ORLAN, 111; forensic facial reconstruction, 164, 170; Neanderthals, 177; face transplant, 222–5, 229

Christianity: the soul, 6; the face in art, 13–14; punishment, 8; physical perfection, 9; influence on sculpture, 11; dissection, 14; stylised portraiture, 14; symbolism, 15; passions, 25; sin, 70; emotional expression, 146

classical sculpture, 5–8

cleft lip, 121, 128

Cleves, Anne of, portrait, 28

clothing: as identity, 16; sumptuary legislation, 53–4; class, 70; fashion and consumer culture, 79–80; New Romantics, 88; influence of cinema, 99

coinage, ruler's faces on, 10–11, 15

colonial contexts, 48, 178; fingerprinting, 61; observations, 84; lingering influence, 110–11

Constantine, Emperor, 11, 14

consumerism: 'selling' the face, 47; consumer goods, 54, 73; focus on appearance, 65, 68; interior design, 76; 'conspicuous consumption', 82–3; manufacturing desire, 83, 98–9; patients as consumers, 97, 105; cosmetic surgery, 101; peer-pressure, 102; choice, 113, 129

corbel heads, 17–18

Cornelius, Robert, 37–40

cosmetics: eighteenth-century, 78–9; gender, 88; market expansion, 98; teaching girls, 131

cosmetic surgery: origins, 91, 99–100; regulation, 97; mental health, 102; bullying, 103; Royal College of Surgeons of England, 104; Eurocentrism, 105; the golden ratio, 109–10, ORLAN, 111; visual social media, 112; the 'uncanny valley', 113

Culp, Connie, 231

cycladic art, 4–5

cynocephaly, *see also* dogs, 13

daguerreotypes, 38, 43–5

Darwin, Charles, 178; 'mirror test', 84–5; *Expression of the Emotions* (1872), 86, 146–8, 150; *On the Origin of Species* (1859), 55, 86

death masks, 46, 160, 238–40

Dee, John, 72

deepfakes, 53, 210

Delacroix, Eugène, *Self-Portrait* (c. 1837), 31

dementia, 206

Descartes, René, 143, 144–55

Devauchelle, Bernard, 222–3

Dickens, Charles, 45–6

Dinoire, Isabelle, 222–7

disfigurement: by disease and punishment, 8–9; definitions of, 103, 121; face transplants, 221 dogs' faces, *see also* cynocephaly *and* animal faces caricature, 13; physiognomy, 7; domestication, 85–6; 'puppy-dog' eyes, 138; speciesism, 139; communication, 199; recognition and smell, 20

donor faces: VCA, 214; matching, 215; transplant, 216; family, 218, 230; as organ, 219; ethics, 221, 231; psychological impact, 224–5; race, 227–8; the language of the gift, 230; prosthetics, 233–5

doppelgängers: Victorian, 51, twins, 52; popular culture, 53; psychological metaphor, 67; in prosopagnosia

Dostoevsky, Fyodor, *The Double*, 52

Down's Syndrome, 129

Dubernard, Jean-Michel, 223

Dubois, Eugène, 166–7

Duchenne, Guillaume, 148–50

Dürer, Albrecht, *Self-Portrait at Twenty-Eight*, 23, 24

Egypt, Fayum mummy portraits, 11–12

Ekman, Paul, *see also* expressions, 151–6

El Jabaly, Yahya ('Boy without a Face'), 120–21

emotions: cultural construction, 154–5; American versus Japanese displays (*see also* Japan), 140, 151; British versus Arabic displays, 155; ethnocentrism and anthropology, 150

Equiano, Olaudah, 28

Este Medical Group, Turkey, 92, 96, 109

Euclid of Alexandria, 6, 107

eugenics, 32, 55, 108

evolution: the face, xx; evolutionary theory, 32, 58, 105, 108, 150–1; appeal of children's faces, 136; visualization, 165; Victorian dioramas, 167, 178–9; adaptation of facial features, 177; archaeological hoaxes, 239–40

expressions: anatomy, xxi, dissection, 5, 14; physiognomy, 7; Roman verism, 9; modern subjectivity, 19; Leonardo, 22; emotions and personality, 25; supplication in servants, 27; complexity in portraiture, 31; early photography, 43–4; facial recognition, 63; in passports, 64; trade in, 98; anatomy, 119 mirroring others 87; facial paralysis, 137; animals, 138–9; pathognomy, 140–41, Le Brun, 142–4; Darwin, 146–9; Freud, 150; cultural differences, 150–52; Ekman's universalism, 151–3; AI, 153; relativism and neuroscience, 154–7; the justice system, 157–8

face transplants: ethical challenges, 226–32; procedure, 215–16; reasons for, 212, 215; standards of care, 218–19; in the UK, 208, 220; world's first procedure (2005), 222–5

face-blindness *see* prosopagnosia

facehood: definition, xix, 2; mirrors, 65; Neanderthals, 182; prosopagnosia, 184; transplants, 207; paradox, 241

facial development, in utero, 119–20

facial paralysis: cosmetic surgery, 104; Moebius Syndrome and Bell's Palsy, 137–8, 140, 156

Index

facial recognition technologies (FRT), and identity, xix; policing and bias, 63–4; in consumer culture, 141

fairy tales: *Snow White*, 88; physical transformations, 94; heroic medical narratives, 223

facial reconstruction, forensic and historical: 3D faces, 160; forensic art, 163–4; in museums, 164–7; influence on historical reconstruction, 167–8; popular culture, 169; Neanderthals, 177–82; Richard III, 173–7; Vasa skeletons, 169–73

facial reconstruction, surgical: origins and Sushruta 100; First and Second World Wars, 101; skin grafts and repair, 101, 213; lip and palate repair, 128; personhood, 168; face transplants, 208, 222

familiar faces: prosopagnosia, 189; emotional connection 191–2; and distinctiveness, 201–3

Fayum mummy portraits, 11–12

fear, *see also* expressions: animal, 138; soul, 141–2; basic emotion, 152; variability, 154–5; amygdala, 190

figurehead, classical purpose, 5, 10; shift away from, 20–21; as symbol, 214, 240

fingerprinting, 61

foetal alcohol syndrome, 132–4

foetal faces: scans, 119, 122; Lennart Nilsson, 123–4; agency to embryos, 125; commercial scans, 128–9; race and racism, 132–5

Freud, Sigmund, 83–4, 101, 150

Galen (Greek physician), 5–6, 59, 138, 142

Galton, Francis, 55–8, 108, 129, 195

gargoyles, 16–18

gender: appearance, 66; cosmetics, 78–9, 87–8, and patriarchy, 90–91; fashion and power, 102; gender affirmation surgery, 104; cosmetic surgery, 112; Galenic theory, 145; emotion, 155–7; science, 170; face transplant, 223; robots, 242

gift, of a face transplant, 212, 230, 232

Gillies, Harold, 101

golden ratio, 6, 19, 106–10

Greece, Ancient, sculpture and physiognomy, 5–8

Guerre, Martin, 50

Gumpp, Johannes, *Triple Self-Portrait*, 80

Gurche, John, 179

Gustav and Gertrude, Vasa Museum, 170–73

Hadid, Bella, 107

Hall of Mirrors, Versailles, 76, 142

Hals, Frans, *The Laughing Cavalier*, 28–9, 29

Harari, Yuval Noah, *Sapiens*, 2

Hardison, Patrick, 231

Hare, William, 14, 118

Henry VIII, 19–20, 22, 28

Herakles (Hercules), 8

Himba (hunter-gatherers in Namibia), 154

His, Wilhelm, Sr, 165

Hitler, Adolf, 108

Holbein, Hans, the Younger: *The Last Supper*, 21; *Portrait of Henry VIII*, 22; *Portrait of Sir Thomas More*, 19–20, 20, 22

Index

homophily, 87
Human Genome Project, and race, 131
humanism, xix, 19, 69, 74, 143
humours, and the humoral, 6–7, 59–60, 142–3, 145
Hunter, William, *The Anatomy of the Gravid Uterus* (1774), 118–19, 122, 124–5, 127

Ibe, Chidiebere, 134–5
Identity: xviii–xxv, historical limits, 3; social meanings, 8, 14, 16; modernity, 33–4; selfies, 41; peasantry, 50; Victorian doppelgängers, 51; passports, 62–3; self-consciousness, 73; consumerism, 83, 98; 'losing face', 140; personhood, 168–9; forensic facial reconstruction, 172; national identity, 177, 183, 240; face transplant, 210–11, 221–44
imago, Roman, 10, 12, 238
individualism: development of, xix, xxiv, 16, 18, 19, 20; formal portraiture, 36; bureaucracy, 50; face as anchor, 51, 54; race, 60; Renaissance, 69, 142; mirrors, 77; foetal, 125; modern, 203, 209
Instagram, *see also* social media: consumer culture, 83; cosmetic surgery, 92, 96–7; 108–11; Australian regulations, 112; homogenization of beauty, 203
intelligence: high forehead, 11, 22; spectacles, 77; expressions, 141, 159; racism and skulls, 165
Interface (project), 109, 208
Inuit, nasal bridge depression, 134
Islam, xxiv, 6, 13, 67

James, William, 150, 155
Japan: 55, 113, 128, 140; facial expression 140, 151, 155, 241; mask-wearing, 156, 224
Java Man ('homo erectus'), 166
Jaw, anatomy, xx, physiognomy, 11, criminals, 59; gender, 104; foetal development, 120–21; forensic facial reconstruction, 163, 168, 170; Neanderthals, 177; Hollywood, 202; face transplants, 216, 234
Jerome, St, 140
Jesus Christ: recognizability, 16; modern image, 18; conception, 115; in Dürer, 23; medieval representation, 119; in pareidolia, 206
Jews and Judaism, idolatry, 13; antisemitism, 45; 108, 136, 182; emotional rituals, 67; legend, 116
Justinian II (Byzantine emperor), 9

Kennis, Adrie and Alfons, the face of Shanidar Z, 162, 179–80
Klein, Naomi, *Doppelganger*, 67
Knox, Amanda, 158

Langley, Philippa, 173, 176–7
Lantieri, Laurent, 213
Lascaux, France, cave paintings in, 3
Lavater, Johann Kaspar, 32, 58, 116, 121, 141
Le Brun, Charles: the science of painting, 25, 143; human emotions, 142–5, 148, influence, 158
Lely, Peter, portraits by, 26
Leng Jun, *Mona Lisa – the Design of a Smile*, 1–2

Index

Leonardo da Vinci: dissection, 14, 18, 23–5; realism, 142; *Mona Lisa*, 21–3, 111; golden ratio, 107, 111
Levinas, Emmanuel, 236, 240
Leviticus, Book of, 121
light, as metaphor, 42; impact on appearance, 43, 68, 82
likeness, and symbolism, 13, 164–5; Anne of Cleves, 28; modern art, 32; photography, 39, 41, 43; forensic facial reconstruction, 175; family resemblance, 230
Linnaeus, Carl, *Systema Naturae*, 48–9, 54, 143, 146
lions: in cave art, 3; physiognomy, 7; anthropomorphic, 17; dissected by Galen, 138
Locke, John, 116
Lombroso, Cesare, criminal faces, 58–9
lorgnettes, 77–8
Lumley, Joanna, 186

Mask of Agamemnon, 238–40, 244
masking, *see also* neurodivergence, 186
masks, social acceptance of, xxiv; *imago*, 10–12; death masks, 36, 160; Oliver Cromwell, 26; ornamental, 30; disfigurement, 103, 122, 212, 224; beauty, 110; pandemic, 122; cultural differences in, 156, 224; prosthetics, 234–5; of Agamemnon, 238; of Tutankhamun, 240; Greek 'persona', 240; Japanese and Greek theatre, 241
McIndoe, Archibald, 101
Mead, Margaret, 150–51
medicine: humoral, 6–7, 142; Chinese 'face reading', 8; head measurements, 122; emotions and the face, 141; the face as organ, 210, 219; racism, 133–4, 141, 227
medieval portraiture: values and traditions, 13, 15–16; declining status, 29
mental health: rising rate of mental illness, 89, 207; consumerism, 99, 207; brain scans and anxiety, 130, 195; pareidolia, 206; modern anxieties about the face and authenticity, 210
Mentsu, the Japanese concept of 'face', 140
micro-expressions, *see also* emotional expression, 139; lying, 152; intuition, 204
Microsoft, emotion-recognition software, 153, 159, 243
mind: relationship to body, xxiii, 59; reflected in Renaissance portraiture, 24; modernity and fragmentation, 33, 207; St Jerome, 140; René Descartes 143–4; expressions, 150; William James, 155; reduction to brain, 187
mirroring behaviour, 86–7
mirrors: Egyptian, 71; European availability, 24, 43, 66, 74–83; Darwin and evolution, 84; Gallup Mirror Test, 85–6; mental health disorders, 89–90; superstitions, 67
Moebius syndrome, 137–8
More, Sir Thomas, 175
Morris, Sir Peter, 220–21
mouches (face patches), 79, 88
Mullins, Joe, 163–4, 168, 171
Munch, Edvard, *The Scream*, 32

Index

muscles and nerves: *see also* anatomy: humans versus primates, xxi, 139; Renaissance dissection, 5, 142; neurofibromatosis, 103; facial nerve development, 119; facial paralysis, 137; electropuncture, 149; marking the skull, 163; forensic facial reconstruction, 164, 179, 180; face transplants, 216, 223, 234, 244

narcissism: Ovid's *Metamorphosis*, 68–70; Caravaggio's *Narcissus at the Fountain*, 69; vanity as sin, 70; Narcissistic Personality Disorder (NPD), 89; mirror use, 90
Neanderthals: communication, 2–3, forensic facial reconstruction, 59, Shanidar Z, 161–3, *162*, 178–82; 'Old Man of La Chapelle', *165*, *166*, 180; and modern humans, 177–9; art and science, 180–82; facial expressions, 181
neurodivergence, 157; and prosopagnosia, 193, 198–9
Newton, Isaac, 76
Nilsson, Lennart, 122–8
Nilsson, Oscar, 170–73
noh (Japanese theatre), use of masks, 241
noses: amputations, 8–9; Oliver Cromwell's nose, 26; antisemitism, 45, 108; Victorian classifications, 49; biometrics, 54; Galton's profiles, 58; Elizabeth I, 72; cosmetics, 87; glabella, 90; cosmetic surgery, 92, 105; Sushruta and surgery, 102; Bella Hadid's nose job, 107; family resemblance, 117, 230–31; born without a nose, 121; Down's Syndrome, 129; Innuit nose bridge, 134; Darwin's nose, 146; gender, 172–3; human evolution, 177

Obsessive-Compulsive Disorder (OCD), *see also* mental health, 89
ORLAN (multimedia artist), 111

Palaeolithic art, 3
pareidolia, 199, 206
Parmigianino, *Self-Portrait in a Convex Mirror*, 74, *75*
Partridge, James, 220–21
passports: conventions, xviii; 34; counterfeit, 53; post-war developments, 61–2; terrorism, 64
pathognomy, 141, 158
Pearson, Adam, 103
Périsset, Jocelyn, 'Bride of Wildenstein', 113
Persian portraiture, 12–13
personhood: the individual, xix; foetal status, 119, 126; empathy, 136, need for a face, 168, 189, 236
philtrum, 115–16, 119–121, 133
photography: camera obscura, 43; *cartes de visite*, 45–7; daguerreotypes, 37–40, 43–5; Kodak camera, 47–8; and light, 42–3; mass surveillance, 61–2; portrait photography, 43–5; post-mortem portraits, 46; selfies, 40–41; to classify, 42, 48–50, 55–60, 80, 209; advertising, 200
physiognomy, 6–7, 15, 30, 32–3, 45, 70, 82, 93, 121; Charles Dickens, 146; and pathognomy, 141, 158
Picasso, Pablo, 5; *The Weeping Woman*, 33

Index

Pitcher, David, 193–6, 197–202
Pitt, Brad, 186, 202–3
Pitt Rivers Museum, Oxford, 167, 184
Poe, Edgar Allan: 'William Wilson', 52, 67; *The Fall of the House of Usher*, 52
Pomahac, Bohdan, *see also* face transplants, 213–17
Pompadour, Madame de, 78, 81
primate faces, *see also* animal faces: facial recognition and the brain, 191, 194; the idea of self, 84–5; expression, 85; the fear/play face, 138; teeth baring, 148
Price, Katie, 113
prosopagnosia, xvii, xxiii, 66, 96, 110, 184; acquired and developmental, 187, 204; brain function, 189–94; neurodivergence, 193, 198–9; place blindness, 187–8; and social context, 192–3, 201–7
prosthetics: Justinian II's gold nose, 9; donor faces, 233–5

race and racism: Linnaeus, 48–9; Meiners, 107; caricatures, 60, 108; Victorian categories, 53; biometrics, 54; eugenics, 57–8; skin tone, 79; photography, 83; cosmetic surgery, 106; beauty, 107; Nazis and the master race, 108; skin whitening, 110; the Other Race Effect, 131–2; Eastern display codes, 140; classifying people, 146; emotional expression, 156; legal system, 158; Human Genomic Project and debunking 'race', 131–2; healthcare, 134, 227, 242; 'scientific' racism, 105, 165;

racism in the museum, 167; association of Black people with Neanderthals, 108, 178, 182; race and technology, 209, modern technology, 243
realism: post-modern hyper-realism, 1; historical significance of, 2, 5; beauty, 6; and verism, 9; medieval irrelevance, 16; Renaissance, 23–4; expression, 30; modernist art, 32, 125; photography, 125
Rejlander, Oscar, 147, 152
Rembrandt, *Portrait of Hermann Doomer*, 25
Renaissance, and European portrait painting, 18–23
Reynolds, Joshua, *Self-Portrait* (c. 1788), 77, 78
Richard III: portraits, 15; facial reconstruction, 161–3, 173–7, 182–3
Robots: 'uncanny valley', 113; eyes and mouths, 179; algorithmic bias, 210; gender, 242; race, 243.
Rococo style, 30–13, 81
Rodriguez, Eduardo, 231, 234
Roentgen, Wilhelm Conrad, 196
Roman portrait statues, 9–10
Romanticism, 31–2
Royal College of Surgeons of England: 14, 94, 104, 220–21, 230
Royal Society for the Prevention of Cruelty to Animals (RSPCA), 139
Rumsey, Nichola, 113
Rymsdyk, Jan van, 118, 125

Sacks, Oliver, 187, 188
Saint Hedwig of Silesia (medieval illumination), 16, 17
Schliemann, Heinrich, 238–40

selfies, 40–41
Severe style, in Ancient Greek art, 5
Shakespeare, William: *Hamlet*, 19; vilification of Richard III, 161, 175
Shanidar Z, *see also* Neanderthals, 161–3, 178–82
Sickle Cell Disease (SCD), 132
Siemionow, Maria, 219, 231, 233
smiling, *see also* expression: in passports, xviii; children's drawings, 1; Leonardo da Vinci, *Mona Lisa*, 22–3, Hals, Franz, *The Laughing Cavalier*, 29, racism and 'watermelon smiles', 55; grooming, 77; Doddy Darwin, 84; cosmetic surgery, 96; emotional labour, 98; baby's preference, 131; dogs smiling, 138; facial paralysis, 140; gender, 156; Neanderthals, 181; technology, 243
social media, *see also* Instagram: 89; cosmetic surgery, 94, 104, 145, 232; filters, 110, 210, 244
social robots, 242–3
statues, facial mutilation, 9
Stevenson, Robert Louis, *The Strange Case of Dr Jekyll and Mr Hyde*, 53
Stubblefield, Katie, 228–30
Super Recognisers International, 189–90
Sushruta (father of surgery), 100

Taylor-Joy, Anya, 107
Tezcatlipoca (Aztec god), 71–2
Tichborne, Roger, 50–51
Toft, Mary, 116–17
Tussaud, Madame, death masks, 160; museum, 183
Tutankhamun, mask of, 240

Underwood, Cameron, 231, 234

Van Eyck, Jan: 25; *The Arnolfini Portrait*, 74, 75
Vasa Museum, 169–70, 172
veil: *Mona Lisa*, 22; the 'Veiled Virgin', 127
Velázquez, Diego Rodriguez de Silva y, *Juan de Pareja* (c. 1650), 27–8, 35
Venice, trade in mirrors, 74–7
Venus of Brassempouy, 1, 3–4
Vergil, Polydore, *Anglica Historia*, 175
Vermeer, Johannes, 24
Vesalius, Andreas, *On the Fabric of the Human Body* (1543), 25, 142
visual impairment: and brain activity, 198; recognising people without sight, 205, 236
vivisection, 84, 138–9

Wiens, Annalyn Bell, 205
Wiens, Dallas, 103
Weston, Simon, 221
whitening creams, *see also* racism, 110
Wilkinson, Caroline, 180; forensic facial reconstruction of Richard III, 162, 164, 175, 183